The Anti-inflammatory Lifestyle diet 2024-2025

*Boost Your Immune System
Naturally Through Diet*

Rhonda C Anderson MS RDN

publisher's or author's permission, you are not allowed to change, distribute, sell, quote from, or paraphrase any part of the book's contents.

Table of Contents

Chapter 1:Understanding Inflammation.

Chapter 2:The Foundation of the Anti-inflammatory Diet.

Chapter 6: Monitoring and Sustaining an Anti-inflammatory Lifestyle.

Chapter 7: Future Trends and Innovations in Anti-inflammatory Living.

7.1 The Latest Research: What Science Says About Inflammation.

7.2 Innovations in Anti-inflammatory Foods and Supplements.

7.3 Tech and Tools: Apps and Gadgets for Health Monitoring.

7.4 Community and Support: Finding Your Tribe.

<u>Disclaimer</u>

Hey there, beautiful soul!

Before you engage or explore into the Anti-inflammatory Lifestyle Diet for 2024-2025, we want to remind you of a few important things. Life can be a journey filled with ups and downs, and we understand that managing inflammation can be incredibly challenging.

This guide is here to support you, offering insights and recommendations that may help you on your path to feeling better. However, everyone's body is unique, and what works for one person might not work for another.

Please, always consult with your healthcare provider before making any significant changes to your diet or lifestyle. They know your medical history and can provide personalised advice tailored to your needs.

Remember, you're not alone in this. We're all in this together, striving for a healthier, happier life. Take each step with kindness towards yourself. Your well-being is a beautiful journey, not a destination.

Stay strong, and take care of yourself. You deserve it!

Dedication

To all the warriors on this journey, this book is dedicated to you—the brave souls who choose to prioritise your health and well-being every single day.

Your strength, resilience, and determination to embrace an anti-inflammatory lifestyle inspire me deeply. Through every challenge and triumph, you demonstrate an unwavering commitment to becoming the best version of yourselves.

Know that you are not alone. Together, we form a community that supports, uplifts, and encourages each other. Each small step you take is a monumental leap toward a healthier, happier life. You are extraordinary, and your journey is a testament to the incredible power within you.

Keep shining, keep believing, and always remember that you are worth every effort. Thank you for being the light that guides and the strength that endures.

With all my heart,

[*Rhonda C Anderson MS RDN*]

Introduction

Welcome **to "The Anti-inflammatory Lifestyle Diet 2024-2025."** This isn't just a book; it's your gateway to a healthier and happier you. We understand that your time is precious, and we are deeply grateful that you've chosen to invest it in reading this book. Rest assured, you've made the right choice. This book is packed with valuable information and practical tips that will transform your diet and, ultimately, your life.

In today's fast-paced world, many of us struggle with inflammation without even realising it. Chronic inflammation can lead to various health issues, including heart disease, diabetes, and arthritis. But the good news is, through thoughtful dietary choices, we can reduce inflammation and improve our overall well-being. "The Anti-inflammatory Lifestyle Diet 2024-2025" offers you the tools and knowledge to take control of your health through food.

What makes this book stand out is its comprehensive approach. Over the years, Rhonda C. Anderson has gained a reputation for creating cookbooks that bring joy and satisfaction to everyone who buys them. Her expertise as a seasoned chef shines through in every recipe and piece of advice she shares. This latest edition is no different. It's designed to guide you every step of the way, ensuring that you get the most out of your investment.

In this book, you'll find a carefully crafted 30-day meal plan. This isn't just any meal plan—it's designed to be easy to follow and enjoyable, making it simple to integrate anti-inflammatory foods into your daily routine. Each recipe has been tested and perfected to ensure it's not only nutritious but also delicious. You won't have to sacrifice taste for health.

Beyond the meal plan, the book includes two other outstanding features: detailed shopping lists and a collection of Rhonda's favourite kitchen tips. These additions are meant to simplify your cooking experience and make it as stress-free as possible. With these tools, you'll be able to shop and cook with confidence, knowing you have everything you need to succeed.

As you read through the pages of this book, you'll gain in-depth knowledge about the foods that can help reduce inflammation and improve your health. You'll learn how to choose the right ingredients, how to prepare them in ways that maximise their health benefits, and how to create meals that your whole family will love.

But knowledge alone isn't enough. The true value of this book comes when you start implementing its advice in your daily life. Follow the step-by-step instructions, try out the recipes, and stick to the meal plan. You'll be amazed at how quickly you start feeling the benefits. Many people across the USA have found joy and improved health through Rhonda's cookbooks, and you're about to join them.

We believe that once you start, you'll not only find the process rewarding but also enjoyable. Cooking doesn't have to be a chore—it can be a delightful experience that brings pleasure and satisfaction. And when you're cooking meals that nourish your body and reduce inflammation, it's even more rewarding.

Thank you for choosing ***"The Anti-inflammatory Lifestyle Diet 2024-2025."*** We're confident that this book will be a valuable addition to your kitchen and a stepping stone to a healthier, more vibrant life. Enjoy every moment, and here's to your health!

Chapter 1:Understanding Inflammation

1.1 The Science of Inflammation: What Is It and Why It Matters

Imagine inflammation like a sizzling pan on the stove. It's your body's way of responding to an injury or threat. Whether it's from a twisted ankle or a pesky cold, inflammation is the body's natural defence mechanism. Let's slice through the layers of what inflammation is and why it's crucial for our health.

What Is Inflammation?

Inflammation is your body's reaction to harm. It's like when you cut your finger chopping vegetables, and it swells up. Your immune system sends a brigade of cells and chemicals to the injured area to fix the problem. These helpers are what cause the swelling, redness, and pain – classic signs of inflammation.

Think of inflammation as a double-edged knife. On one hand, it's essential for healing. Without it, even minor injuries could become major problems. On the other hand, if inflammation lingers, it can cause damage, like leaving the stove on too long and burning the dish.

Why Inflammation Matters

Understanding inflammation is like knowing your ingredients in cooking. It's fundamental to managing your health and preventing disease. Here's why it matters:

1.Healing and Repair: Inflammation is crucial for healing wounds and fighting off infections. It's like the emergency responders of your body, rushing to the scene to provide aid.

2.Chronic Diseases: Persistent inflammation can lead to or worsen chronic conditions. Imagine if your pan continues to overheat – eventually, it damages whatever is in it. The same goes for your body. Chronic inflammation can contribute to conditions like Alzheimer's, cancer, and asthma.

3.Immune System: Your immune system relies on inflammation to protect you. However, if it's always on high alert, it can start attacking healthy tissues, leading to autoimmune diseases.

4.Lifestyle Impact: Your lifestyle choices, like diet, exercise, and stress levels, can influence inflammation. Eating a balanced diet, staying active, and managing stress are like using the right amount of heat in cooking – they keep inflammation under control.

<u>Managing Inflammation</u>

Keeping inflammation in check is like mastering the art of cooking. It requires a balanced approach:

<u>1.Eat a Healthy Diet:</u> Fill your plate with a variety of whole foods, focusing on fruits, vegetables, and lean proteins. Avoid processed foods and added sugars as much as possible.

<u>2.Stay Active:</u> Regular exercise helps keep inflammation levels in check. It's like stirring the pot – it keeps things moving and prevents burning.

<u>3.Get Enough Sleep:</u> Rest is crucial for recovery and managing inflammation. It's like letting your pan cool down after cooking.

<u>4.Manage Stress:</u> High stress can fuel chronic inflammation. Practices like meditation, yoga, or even a walk can help keep your stress levels and inflammation low.

1.2 Chronic vs. Acute Inflammation: Key Differences

Acute Inflammation

is short-term. It's like a quick boil on the stove. This happens when you sprain your ankle or get a bug bite. Your body jumps into action, deals with the issue, and then cools down. This type of inflammation is generally good – it means your body is healing.

Chronic Inflammation

 is more like a slow simmer that never stops. It occurs when the body continues to send inflammatory responses even when there's no immediate injury or threat. This can happen due to persistent issues like stress, poor diet, or autoimmune diseases. Over time, chronic inflammation can lead to serious health problems, like heart disease, diabetes, or arthritis.

1.3 Health Implications: From Arthritis to Heart Disease

1.4 The Role of Diet in Inflammation

Just like the ingredients you choose in cooking affect the flavour of your dish, your diet plays a huge role in inflammation. Some foods can increase inflammation, while others can help reduce it.

<u>Pro-Inflammatory Foods:</u> These are like adding too much salt to a dish. Foods high in sugar, refined carbs, and unhealthy fats can trigger inflammation. Think of sugary drinks, white bread, and fried foods.

<u>Anti-Inflammatory Foods:</u> These are the fresh herbs and spices that bring balance to your meal. Fruits, vegetables, nuts, fatty fish, and olive oil can help reduce inflammation. They are rich in antioxidants and healthy fats, which are like the cooling agents to an overheated pan.

1.5.Assessing Your Inflammatory Health: Self-Evaluation and Testing

Signs You Might Have Chronic Inflammation

Recognizing chronic inflammation isn't always straightforward. Here are some signs you might notice:

1.*Persistent Fatigue:* Feeling constantly tired, even after a good night's sleep.

2.Joint Pain: Aching or stiff joints without a clear cause.

3.Digestive Issues: Problems like bloating, diarrhoea, or constipation that don't seem to go away.

4.Skin Problems: Rashes, eczema, or other skin irritations.

5.Weight Fluctuations: Gaining or losing weight unexpectedly.

6.Frequent Infections: Getting sick more often than usual.

These symptoms can be clues that something is off with your body's inflammation levels.

Self-Evaluation Tips

Before running to the doctor, you can take some steps at home to assess your inflammation. Here's how:

1.Keep a Journal: Write down your daily energy levels, pain, and other symptoms. Look for patterns over time.

2.Check Your Diet: Are you eating a lot of processed foods, sugar, or unhealthy fats? These can fuel inflammation.

3.Monitor Your Stress: Notice how often you feel stressed and what triggers it. Stress can increase inflammation in your body.

4.Assess Your Sleep: Are you getting 7-9 hours of good sleep each night? Poor sleep can contribute to inflammation.

5.Move More: See if you're getting enough physical activity. Regular exercise can help reduce inflammation.

Tests to Measure Inflammation

If your self-evaluation suggests you might have chronic inflammation, the next step is to get some tests. Here are the most common ones:

1.C-Reactive Protein (CRP) Test: This blood test measures the level of CRP, a protein made by your liver. High levels of CRP indicate inflammation.

2.Erythrocyte Sedimentation Rate (ESR) Test: Also a blood test, this one checks how quickly red blood cells settle at the bottom of a test tube. Faster settling can mean more inflammation.

3.Fibrinogen Test: Fibrinogen is a blood clotting protein. High levels can point to inflammation.

4.Homocysteine Test: This measures the level of homocysteine, an amino acid. High levels are linked to inflammation and heart disease.

5.Blood Sugar Tests: High blood sugar levels can lead to inflammation, so testing your glucose can be informative.

How to Reduce Inflammation

If you find out that you have high inflammation, don't worry. There are plenty of ways to reduce it. Here's what you can do:

1.Eat Anti-Inflammatory Foods: Focus on fruits, vegetables, nuts, and fatty fish like salmon. Avoid processed foods and sugar.

2.Exercise Regularly: Aim for at least 30 minutes of moderate exercise most days.

3.Manage Stress: Try activities like yoga, meditation, or deep breathing to help keep stress levels in check.

4.Get Enough Sleep: Stick to a regular sleep schedule and make your bedroom a restful place.

5.Quit Smoking: Smoking is a major cause of inflammation. If you smoke, seek help to quit.

When to See a Doctor

While self-assessment and lifestyle changes are powerful tools, it's important to seek medical advice if you have persistent symptoms or if your self-evaluation points to chronic inflammation. A healthcare professional can guide you through more detailed testing and treatment options.

Keeping your body's inflammation in check is like maintaining a well-tuned kitchen. When everything is in balance, you feel great and can cook up a storm. But when inflammation gets out of hand, it's like a kitchen fire that needs to be put out quickly to prevent further damage.

By understanding and managing your inflammation, you can keep your body healthy and your "kitchen" running smoothly.

Chapter 2:The Foundation of the Anti-inflammatory Diet

2.1.Principles of Anti-inflammatory Eating

Focus on Whole Foods

First and foremost, choose whole foods. Think fresh fruits, vegetables, whole grains, and lean proteins. These foods are packed with nutrients and have minimal processing, making them rich in natural goodness. Fresh produce like berries, leafy greens, and bell peppers are not only colorful and delicious but also loaded with antioxidants that combat inflammation.

Whole grains such as brown rice, quinoa, and oats provide fiber, which helps maintain a healthy gut. A healthy gut is crucial because it's linked to reduced inflammation throughout the body. Lean proteins, including fish, poultry, beans, and nuts, are essential as they supply amino acids necessary for repair and growth without the added burden of saturated fats found in processed meats.

Prioritize Healthy Fats

Fats often get a bad rap, but not all fats are created equal. Healthy fats, like those found in olive oil, avocados, and nuts, are excellent for fighting inflammation. Omega-3 fatty acids, in particular, are superstar fats. You can find them in fatty fish like salmon, mackerel, and sardines. These fats help reduce the production of inflammatory compounds and support heart health.

In contrast, try to cut down on trans fats and saturated fats found in fried foods, pastries, and processed snacks. These fats can trigger inflammation and are linked to various chronic diseases.

Spice It Up

Spices are more than just flavor enhancers—they are powerful anti-inflammatory agents. Turmeric, with its active compound curcumin, is a potent anti-inflammatory. You can add it to soups, stews, and even smoothies. Ginger is another spice that's great for reducing inflammation and can be used in teas, marinades, and dressings.

Garlic and cinnamon are also excellent choices. Garlic contains sulfur compounds that activate the immune system, while cinnamon helps regulate blood sugar levels, reducing inflammation.

Limit Added Sugars

Sugar is a major player in the inflammation game. Too much of it can spike blood sugar levels, leading to an inflammatory response. Opt for natural sweeteners like honey or maple syrup in moderation, and try to satisfy your sweet tooth with fruits, which come with fiber and vitamins that help mitigate sugar's impact on inflammation.

Avoid sugary drinks, candies, and baked goods that are loaded with refined sugars. Reading labels is key—look out for hidden sugars in products that might not taste particularly sweet, like sauces and dressings.

Stay Hydrated

Water is essential for every function in our bodies, including reducing inflammation. Staying well-hydrated helps flush toxins out of the body and keeps our joints lubricated, reducing pain and stiffness. Aim for at least eight glasses of water a day, and consider green tea, which is rich in anti-inflammatory compounds, as an additional hydration source.

Eat a Rainbow

Variety is the spice of life, and it's also a cornerstone of anti-inflammatory eating. Each colour in fruits and vegetables represents different phytonutrients that fight inflammation in various ways. For example, red tomatoes contain lycopene, while orange carrots are rich in beta-carotene. Aiming to fill your plate with a rainbow of colours ensures you're getting a broad spectrum of nutrients that work together to combat inflammation.

Balance and Moderation

It's important to remember that anti-inflammatory eating doesn't mean deprivation. It's about balance and making smarter choices. You don't have to give up all your favourite foods; just try to enjoy them in moderation. Swap out less healthy options for more nutritious ones when possible, and don't beat yourself up if you indulge occasionally.

Listen to Your Body

Every person is different, and what works for one might not work for another. Pay attention to how different foods make you feel. If something causes discomfort or seems to trigger inflammation, try eliminating it and see how you respond. Keeping a food diary can be helpful in identifying patterns and understanding your body's unique needs.

2.2 Essential Nutrients and Their Anti-inflammatory Roles

Omega-3 Fatty Acids: The Soothing Fats

Omega-3 fatty acids are found in fatty fish like salmon, mackerel, and sardines, as well as in flaxseeds, chia seeds, and walnuts. These healthy fats are like the calming agents of our diet. They help reduce inflammation by blocking the production of substances that promote it. Think of them as the firefighters who rush in to calm things down.

Including omega-3-rich foods in your diet can help lower the risk of chronic diseases such as heart disease and arthritis. They can also boost your mood and cognitive function. So, when you're grilling up some fish or sprinkling seeds on your salad, you're doing more than adding flavor—you're nourishing your body with powerful anti-inflammatory agents.

Antioxidants: The Body's Defense System

Antioxidants are compounds found in colorful fruits and vegetables like berries, spinach, and bell peppers. They protect our cells from damage caused by free radicals, which are unstable molecules that can cause inflammation. Imagine antioxidants as a shield that guards your body against harmful invaders.

Vitamins A, C, and E, as well as minerals like selenium and zinc, are potent antioxidants. They help reduce oxidative stress, which is a key factor in chronic inflammation. Including a rainbow of fruits and vegetables in your diet ensures that you're getting a variety of antioxidants to keep inflammation at bay.

Fiber: The Gentle Cleanser

Fiber is found in whole grains, fruits, vegetables, and legumes. It's like a gentle broom that sweeps through your digestive system, keeping everything moving smoothly. But fiber does more than just support digestion; it also feeds the beneficial bacteria in your gut, which play a crucial role in managing inflammation.

A healthy gut is essential for a strong immune system. When your gut bacteria are well-fed, they produce substances that help control inflammation throughout your body. Aim for a variety of fiber-rich foods to support a healthy gut and a well-balanced immune response.

Polyphenols: The Plant Protectors

Polyphenols are compounds found in plant foods like green tea, olive oil, dark chocolate, and many fruits and vegetables. These nutrients are like the protectors of the plant world, and they offer the same benefits to us. They help reduce inflammation and support overall health.

Green tea, for example, is rich in a type of polyphenol called catechins, which have powerful anti-inflammatory effects. Similarly, the polyphenols in olive oil can help reduce markers of inflammation in the body. Adding a splash of olive oil to your salads or enjoying a cup of green tea can be a simple yet effective way to combat inflammation.

Vitamin D: The Sunshine Vitamin

Vitamin D, often known as the sunshine vitamin, is crucial for immune function and inflammation control. Our bodies produce vitamin D when we're exposed to sunlight, but it can also be found in foods like fatty fish, fortified dairy products, and eggs.

Vitamin D helps regulate the immune system and can reduce the production of inflammatory substances in the body. Low levels of vitamin D have been linked to an increased risk of inflammatory diseases. Ensuring adequate exposure to sunlight and consuming vitamin D-rich foods can help keep inflammation under control.

Probiotics: The Friendly Bacteria

Probiotics are beneficial bacteria found in fermented foods like yogurt, kefir, sauerkraut, and kimchi. They are like the friendly neighbors who help keep your gut community balanced and healthy. A well-balanced gut microbiome can reduce inflammation and support overall health.

Including a variety of probiotic-rich foods in your diet can help maintain a healthy gut, which in turn can reduce systemic inflammation. So, the next time you reach for that bowl of yogurt or a serving of kimchi, remember that you're nurturing your body's natural defenses against inflammation.

2.3.Superfoods to Fight Inflammation

1.Turmeric

Turmeric is more than just a bright yellow spice used in curries. It's packed with curcumin, a powerful anti-inflammatory compound. Curcumin can help reduce inflammation at the molecular level. To get the most out of turmeric, combine it with black pepper, which enhances the absorption of curcumin. Try adding a pinch to soups, smoothies, or even tea for a flavorful, anti-inflammatory boost.

2.Ginger

Ginger, a close relative of turmeric, is another potent anti-inflammatory agent. It contains gingerol, which has been shown to reduce inflammation and muscle pain. Fresh ginger can add a zesty kick to stir-fries, soups, and marinades. For a soothing option, brew a cup of ginger tea with a slice of lemon and honey.

3.Berries

Berries are tiny powerhouses of antioxidants, which help fight inflammation. Blueberries, strawberries, raspberries, and blackberries are rich in anthocyanins, compounds that reduce inflammation and oxidative stress. They're perfect for snacking, adding to cereal, or blending into a vibrant smoothie.

4.Fatty Fish

Fatty fish like salmon, mackerel, and sardines are high in omega-3 fatty acids, which have strong anti-inflammatory properties. These healthy fats can help reduce the risk of heart disease and lower inflammation levels in the body. For a delicious and healthy meal, bake or grill fish and serve it with a fresh salad or steamed vegetables.

5.Green Leafy Vegetables

Spinach, kale, and Swiss chard are rich in vitamins, minerals, and antioxidants that combat inflammation. They're also high in fiber, which promotes a healthy gut. Enjoy them in salads, smoothies, or lightly sautéed with garlic and olive oil for a quick and nutritious side dish.

6.Nuts and Seeds

Nuts and seeds, like almonds, walnuts, chia seeds, and flaxseeds, are excellent sources of healthy fats, protein, and fiber. They also contain magnesium, which has been linked to reduced inflammation. Sprinkle them on yogurt, salads, or oatmeal, or enjoy them as a snack to keep inflammation at bay.

7.Olive Oil

Extra virgin olive oil is a staple of the Mediterranean diet and is well-known for its anti-inflammatory benefits. It's rich in oleocanthal, a compound with similar effects to ibuprofen in reducing inflammation. Use olive oil as a base for salad dressings, drizzle it over cooked vegetables, or dip whole-grain bread into it for a simple yet delicious appetizer.

8.Garlic

Garlic has been used for its medicinal properties for centuries. It contains sulfur compounds, like allicin, which help reduce inflammation. Garlic adds a robust flavor to dishes and can be used in a variety of ways – from roasting whole cloves to adding minced garlic to sauces and dressings.

9.Green Tea

Green tea is loaded with antioxidants, particularly catechins, which have anti-inflammatory effects. Drinking green tea regularly can help reduce inflammation and protect against cell damage. Enjoy a cup in the morning or as an afternoon pick-me-up.

10.Tomatoes

Tomatoes are a great source of lycopene, an antioxidant with powerful anti-inflammatory properties. Cooking tomatoes increases the lycopene content, making tomato-based sauces and soups excellent choices. Add fresh tomatoes to salads, sandwiches, or enjoy them roasted with a sprinkle of herbs.

2.4 Foods to Avoid: The Inflammatory Culprits

1.Refined Sugars and High-Fructose Corn Syrup

Refined sugars are found in sodas, candy, baked goods, and even some savory items. These sugars spike blood glucose levels, leading to an inflammatory response. High-fructose corn syrup, a common sweetener in processed foods, is particularly harmful. It's found in many soft drinks and packaged snacks.

Better Choices: Opt for natural sweeteners like honey, maple syrup, or stevia. They're less processed and used in moderation, they don't cause the same spikes in blood sugar.

2.Trans Fats

Trans fats are artificial fats created during food processing to extend shelf life. They're found in margarine, fast foods, and many packaged baked goods. Trans fats not only raise bad cholesterol levels but also trigger inflammation, increasing the risk of heart disease.

Better Choices: Use healthier fats like olive oil, avocado oil, or coconut oil for cooking and baking. Natural sources of fats, such as nuts, seeds, and fatty fish like salmon, are also excellent options.

3.Refined Carbohydrates

White bread, white rice, and most pastries fall under refined carbohydrates. They are stripped of nutrients and fiber during processing. These foods are quickly digested, causing a rapid increase in blood sugar and, subsequently, inflammation.

Better Choices: Whole grains like brown rice, quinoa, and whole wheat bread are rich in nutrients and fibre, providing a slower, more steady release of glucose into the bloodstream.

4.Processed Meats

Processed meats such as bacon, sausages, and deli meats contain preservatives and other additives that can provoke inflammation. These meats often have high levels of salt and unhealthy fats, contributing further to the problem.

Better Choices: Choose fresh, lean meats and poultry. If you enjoy cured meats, look for options with minimal processing and no added nitrates or nitrites. Consider plant-based proteins like beans, lentils, and tofu as healthy alternatives.

5.Excessive Alcohol

While moderate alcohol consumption, especially red wine, might offer some health benefits, excessive drinking can lead to severe inflammation. Alcohol affects the liver and other organs, and over time, it can cause inflammation throughout the body.

Better Choices: Drink alcohol in moderation. If you enjoy a glass of wine or beer, keep it to a reasonable limit, such as one drink per day for women and two for men. Consider non-alcoholic beverages, like herbal teas or sparkling water with a splash of fruit juice, for a refreshing alternative.

6. Artificial Additives

Many processed foods contain artificial additives, including colours, flavours, and preservatives. These additives can irritate the body and promote inflammation, especially in individuals with sensitivities or allergies.

Better Choices: Stick to whole, unprocessed foods whenever possible. When buying packaged items, read labels carefully and choose products with few and recognizable ingredients. Fresh fruits, vegetables, and home-cooked meals are often the safest bet.

7. Excess Omega-6 Fatty Acids

Omega-6 fatty acids are essential fats found in many vegetable oils like corn oil, soybean oil, and sunflower oil. While they are necessary for health, too much omega-6 and not enough omega-3 can lead to an imbalance that promotes inflammation.

Better Choices: Balance your intake by incorporating more omega-3 rich foods, such as fish, chia seeds, and walnuts. Use oils like olive oil or avocado oil, which have a healthier fatty acid profile.

Chapter 3: Personalised Anti-inflammatory Plans

3.1 Tailoring the Diet to Your Needs: Age, Gender, and Lifestyle

Age Matters

For Children and Teens:

Growing bodies need plenty of nutrients, and kids often face different dietary challenges. Focus on colorful fruits and veggies like berries and carrots, which are high in antioxidants. Whole grains like oats and quinoa provide steady energy and fiber. It's also important to include healthy fats from fish or avocados, which support brain development. Keep an eye on sugar and processed foods, as they can spike inflammation and energy levels.

For Adults in Their 20s to 40s:

This is the time to set the foundation for long-term health. Incorporate a variety of leafy greens, lean proteins like chicken or tofu, and nuts or seeds for healthy fats. At this stage, it's also about balancing work, family, and personal time, which can be stressful. Foods rich in omega-3 fatty acids, such as salmon or flaxseeds, help combat stress and inflammation. Keep hydrated and watch caffeine and alcohol intake, which can contribute to inflammation if consumed in excess.

For Adults Over 50:

As you age, maintaining muscle mass and bone health becomes crucial. Calcium and vitamin D are essential, so include dairy or fortified alternatives. Lean proteins, like beans or fish, support muscle health. Fiber-rich foods like whole grains and fruits aid digestion and help manage weight. Inflammation often increases with age, so focusing on anti-inflammatory spices like turmeric and ginger can be beneficial. Staying active and engaging in low-impact exercises like walking or swimming can also help reduce inflammation.

Gender Differences

For Women:

Women have unique nutritional needs, especially concerning hormonal changes. Foods high in phytoestrogens, like flaxseeds and soy, can help balance hormones. Iron-rich foods, such as spinach and legumes, are crucial, especially during menstruation. For those going through menopause, incorporating calcium-rich foods helps maintain bone health. Omega-3 fatty acids found in fish can ease menstrual cramps and reduce inflammation.

For Men:

Men often require more calories and protein to maintain muscle mass. Lean meats, fish, and legumes are excellent choices. Zinc-rich foods, like pumpkin seeds and nuts, support immune health and testosterone production. Reducing red meat and processed foods can lower the risk of heart disease and inflammation. Including cruciferous vegetables, like broccoli and Brussels sprouts, can help protect against certain cancers common in men.

Tailoring to Your Lifestyle

Active Individuals and Athletes:

If you're regularly active or an athlete, your body has increased needs for nutrients and calories. Carbohydrates from whole grains, fruits, and vegetables provide the necessary fuel. Protein is essential for muscle recovery and should come from lean sources like chicken, fish, or plant-based options. Healthy fats from avocados, nuts, and olive oil help reduce inflammation and support overall energy levels. Hydration is key, so drink plenty of water and consider electrolyte-rich drinks if you sweat a lot.

Busy Professionals:

For those constantly on the go, planning is crucial. Meal prepping with anti-inflammatory staples like quinoa salads, grilled chicken, and roasted veggies can save time and keep you on track. Snacking on nuts, seeds, or fresh fruit instead of processed snacks helps keep inflammation at bay. Staying hydrated and taking breaks to stretch or move can reduce stress and support overall well-being.

Elders and Those with Chronic Conditions:

For older adults or those dealing with chronic health issues, focus on nutrient-dense, easy-to-digest foods. Soups made with vegetables and lean proteins can be soothing and nutritious. Incorporate anti-inflammatory herbs and spices, like turmeric and ginger, into meals. Regular, gentle activity like tai chi or yoga can aid digestion and reduce inflammation.

3.2 Anti-inflammatory Diet for Athletes

As athletes, maintaining peak performance and swift recovery is crucial. What you eat plays a huge role in managing inflammation, which is a natural response to intense training but can become a problem if it's chronic. By choosing the right foods, you can help your body recover faster and stay in top shape. Let's dive into how an anti-inflammatory diet can be a game-changer for athletes.

Understanding Inflammation and Its Impact

Inflammation is your body's way of protecting itself. After a tough workout, your muscles experience tiny tears. In response, your body sends in white blood cells to repair the damage, causing temporary inflammation. This process is essential for muscle growth and adaptation. However, when inflammation lingers or becomes chronic, it can lead to pain, fatigue, and even long-term health issues. This is where an anti-inflammatory diet comes in, helping to keep inflammation at healthy levels and supporting overall well-being.

Meal Ideas for Athletes

To give you a practical guide, here are some meal ideas that fit perfectly into an anti-inflammatory diet:

Breakfast: Start your day with a bowl of oatmeal topped with berries, chia seeds, and a drizzle of honey. Add a side of green tea.

Lunch: Enjoy a quinoa salad with mixed greens, cherry tomatoes, avocado, grilled chicken, and a lemon-turmeric vinaigrette.

Dinner: Savour grilled salmon with a side of steamed broccoli and sweet potato wedges. Season with garlic and olive oil.

Snacks: Keep it simple with apple slices and almond butter or a handful of mixed nuts.

The Benefits of an Anti-Inflammatory Diet

For athletes, the advantages are clear. An anti-inflammatory diet can help reduce muscle soreness, speed up recovery, and improve overall performance. It also supports heart health, enhances brain function, and helps maintain a healthy weight. By making thoughtful food choices, you can help your body stay strong and resilient, ready to tackle the next challenge.

3.3.Managing Chronic Conditions: Diabetes, Autoimmune Diseases, and More

1.*Diabetes Management:* For those with diabetes, maintaining stable blood sugar levels is crucial. An anti-inflammatory diet helps by including foods that have a low glycemic index, meaning they don't cause spikes in blood sugar. Foods like whole grains, vegetables, and lean proteins are all good choices.

2.*Autoimmune Diseases:* Conditions like rheumatoid arthritis, lupus, and multiple sclerosis involve the immune system attacking the body. By reducing inflammation through diet, symptoms like pain and fatigue can often be managed better. Omega-3 fatty acids, found in fatty fish and flaxseeds, are particularly beneficial for reducing inflammation in autoimmune diseases.

3.Heart Health: Chronic inflammation can contribute to heart disease. An anti-inflammatory diet rich in fruits, vegetables, and healthy fats can help protect the heart by reducing the levels of bad cholesterol and keeping blood vessels healthy.

3.4 Weight Management with Anti-inflammatory Foods

1.Reducing Inflammation: Chronic inflammation can lead to weight gain. By eating anti-inflammatory foods, you help your body combat this inflammation, making it easier to maintain a healthy weight.

2.Improving Digestion: Many anti-inflammatory foods are high in fiber, which supports healthy digestion. A well-functioning digestive system helps in the efficient breakdown of food and absorption of nutrients, preventing the build-up of toxins and fat.

3.Balancing Blood Sugar Levels: Foods like whole grains, nuts, and leafy greens help stabilize your blood sugar. This prevents spikes and crashes that can lead to overeating and weight gain.

4.Boosting Metabolism: Foods rich in omega-3 fatty acids, such as fish and flaxseeds, can help boost your metabolism, aiding in weight loss.

5.Promoting Satiety: High-fiber foods and healthy fats keep you feeling full longer. This helps prevent overeating and the temptation to reach for unhealthy snacks.

Practical Tips for Incorporating Anti-inflammatory Foods

1.Start Small: Add a serving of fruits or vegetables to each meal. Snack on nuts or seeds instead of chips or candy.

2.Swap Ingredients: Replace refined grains with whole grains. Use olive oil instead of butter or margarine.

3.Spice It Up: Add herbs and spices to your dishes. Not only do they enhance flavor, but they also boost your health.

4.Plan Your Meals: Preparing your meals in advance can help you avoid unhealthy choices. Include a mix of anti-inflammatory foods to keep your diet varied and enjoyable.

5.Stay Hydrated: Drink plenty of water and include herbal teas in your daily routine.

3.5 Anti-inflammatory Diet for Families: From Kids to Seniors

Anti-inflammatory Foods

Choosing the right foods is key to reducing inflammation. Here's a breakdown of what to include in your diet:

1.*Fruits and Vegetables:* These are rich in antioxidants and nutrients. Berries, leafy greens, tomatoes, and avocados are all great choices. Aim to fill half your plate with fruits and veggies at each meal.

2.*Whole Grains:* Brown rice, quinoa, oats, and whole wheat are full of fibre, which can help lower inflammation. Swap out white bread and pasta for their whole-grain versions.

3.*Healthy Fats:* Fats from fish like salmon, nuts, seeds, and olive oil are beneficial. They contain omega-3 fatty acids, which are known to reduce inflammation.

4.Lean Proteins: Choose proteins like chicken, turkey, and plant-based options like beans and lentils. These are easier on the body compared to processed meats.

5.Spices and Herbs: Turmeric, ginger, garlic, and cinnamon not only add flavour but also have powerful anti-inflammatory properties.

Foods to Limit

Just as some foods help fight inflammation, others can make it worse. It's best to limit:

1.Sugary Foods and Drinks: Sweets, sodas, and even fruit juices can spike your blood sugar and increase inflammation.

2.Processed Foods: Items like chips, cookies, and frozen meals often contain unhealthy fats and additives that can lead to inflammation.

3.Red and Processed Meats: Too much red meat or processed meat can contribute to inflammation and other health problems.

4.Refined Carbs: White bread, white rice, and pastries can increase blood sugar and inflammation.

5.Excessive Alcohol: While moderate drinking might be okay, too much alcohol can lead to inflammation and other health issues.

Meal Planning for Families

Creating a meal plan that suits everyone in the family can be fun and rewarding. Here are some tips to get started:

1.Include Everyone: Ask family members about their favourite healthy foods and try to include them in your meal plan. This makes meals enjoyable for everyone.

2.Make it Colourful: Use a variety of fruits and vegetables to keep meals interesting. The more colours on your plate, the more nutrients you're getting.

3.Cook Together: Involve kids in cooking. They're more likely to eat what they help prepare. It's also a great way to teach them about healthy eating.

4.Batch Cooking: Prepare larger portions of meals that can be stored and used later in the week. This saves time and ensures you always have something healthy on hand.

5.Healthy Snacks: Keep snacks like nuts, yoghurt, fruits, and veggies ready to go. These are much better options than chips or candy.

Eating Out and Special Occasions

Eating out or attending special events doesn't mean you have to abandon your anti-inflammatory diet. Here's how to stay on track:

1.Choose Wisely: Look for menu items that include lots of vegetables, lean proteins, and whole grains. Ask for dressings and sauces on the side to control how much you consume.

2.Portion Control: Restaurants often serve large portions. Consider sharing a dish or saving half for later.

3.Enjoy Treats in Moderation: It's okay to have treats occasionally. Just be mindful of portion sizes and try to balance them with healthier choices throughout the day.

Chapter 4: Recipes to Reduce Inflammation

4.1 Breakfasts that Kickstart Healing.

1.Almond Berry Smoothie

Prep Time:10 mins
Total Time:10 mins
Serving:1

Ingredients

- 1 cup frozen blueberries
- 1 banana
- ½ cup almond milk
- 1 tablespoon almond butter
- water as needed

Directions.

1.Combine blueberries, a banana, almond milk, and almond butter in a blender. Blend until the mixture is smooth, adding water if you prefer a thinner consistency.

Nutritional value
Carbs:56g
Protein:7g
Calories:321
Fat:14g

2.Strawberry Rhubarb Crisp

Prep Time:15 mins
Cook Time:45 mins
Total Time:1 hr
Serving:12.

Ingredients

Fruit Layer:

- 3 cups sliced fresh strawberries
- 3 cups diced rhubarb
- 1 cup white sugar
- 3 tablespoons all-purpose flour

Crunch Topping:

- 1 ½ cups all-purpose flour
- 1 cup packed brown sugar
- 1 cup rolled oats
- 1 cup butter

Directions.

1. Gather all the ingredients.

2. Preheat your oven to 375°F (190°C).

3. Prepare the fruit layer by mixing strawberries, rhubarb, white sugar, and flour in a large bowl. Spread this mixture evenly in a 9x13-inch baking dish.

4. For the topping, blend 1 ½ cups of flour, brown sugar, oats, and butter until the mixture is crumbly. A pastry cutter can be helpful for this step. Sprinkle the topping over the fruit layer.

5. Bake in the preheated oven until the topping is crisp and golden brown, about 45 minutes.

6. Serve and enjoy!

<u>Nutritional value</u>
Carbs:54g
Protein:4g
Calories:368
Fat:19g

3.Healthy Berry and Spinach Smoothie.

Prep Time:10 mins
Total Time:10 mins

Serving:4

Ingredients

- 2 cups frozen berries
- 1 cup plain yoghourt
- ½ cup orange juice
- ¼ cup fresh spinach, or to taste
- 5 strawberries

Directions.

1.Combine berries, yoghourt, orange juice, spinach, and strawberries in a blender and blend until smooth.

Nutritional value
Carbs:18g
Protein:4g
Calories:88
Fat:21g

4.Creamy Avocado Egg Salad.

Prep Time:15 mins
Total Time:15 mins
Serving:6

<u>Ingredients</u>

- 6 hard-cooked eggs, chopped
- 2 large avocados, peeled and chopped
- 1 cup seeded and chopped tomatoes
- ½ cup diced red onion
- salt and ground black pepper to taste
- 2 tablespoons mayonnaise
- 2 tablespoons sour cream
- 1 tablespoon lemon juice
- 10 drops hot sauce (such as Frank's RedHot ®)

<u>Directions.</u>

1.In a bowl, mix together eggs, avocados, tomatoes, and red onion, seasoning with salt and pepper. Add mayonnaise, sour cream, lemon juice, and hot sauce to the mixture and stir until everything is well combined.

Nutritional value
Carbs:12g
Protein:9g
Calories:284
Fat:30g

5.Green Smoothie.

Prep Time:10
Total Time:
Serving:

Ingredients

- 1 banana, cut in chunks
- 1 cup grapes
- 1 (6 ounce) tub vanilla yoghourt
- ½ apple, cored and chopped
- 1 ½ cups fresh spinach leaves

Directions.

Add the banana, grapes, yogurt, apple, and spinach to the blender. Cover and blend until the mixture is smooth, occasionally pausing to scrape down the sides. Pour into glasses and enjoy.

Nutritional value

Carbs:45g
Protein:6g
Calories:205
Fat:2g

6.Kale and Banana Smoothie

Prep Time:5 mins

Total Time:5 mins
Serving:1

Ingredients

- 2 cups chopped kale
- 1 banana
- ½ cup light unsweetened soy milk
- 1 tablespoon flax seeds
- 1 teaspoon maple syrup

Directions.

1. Assemble all the ingredients.

2. Add the kale, banana, soy milk, flax seeds, and maple syrup to a blender.

3. Blend until the mixture is smooth.

4. Pour the smoothie over ice and serve.

Nutritional value
Carbs:57g
Protein:15g

Calories:318
Fat:8g

7.Avocado, Blueberry, Banana, and Chia Smoothie.

Prep Time:10 mins
Total Time:10 mins
Serving:1

<u>Ingredients</u>

- 1 cup vanilla-flavoured almond milk
- 1 avocado - peeled, pitted, and halved
- 1 cup fresh blueberries
- 1 banana
- 1 cup ice
- 1 tablespoon chia seeds

Directions.

1.In a blender, mix almond milk, avocado, blueberries, banana, ice, and chia seeds; blend until the mixture is smooth.

Nutritional value
Carbs:86g
Protein:9g
Calories:645
Fat:35g

8.Purple Monstrosity Fruit Smoothie

Prep Time:5 mins
Total Time:5 mins
Serving:5.

Ingredients

- 2 frozen bananas, skins removed and cut in chunks

- ½ cup frozen blueberries
- 1 cup orange juice
- 1 tablespoon honey (Optional)
- 1 teaspoon vanilla extract (Optional

Directions.

1.Combine bananas, blueberries, and juice in a blender, and blend until smooth. Adjust the sweetness with honey or vanilla as desired. Add more or less liquid to achieve your preferred smoothie consistency.

Nutritional value
Carbs:21g
Protein:1g
Calories:88
Fat:0g

9.Chocolate Raspberry Chia Parfaits.

Prep Time:10 mins
Chill Time:30 mins
Total Time:40 mins
Serving:2

Ingredients
Chia Pudding:
- 3/4 cup Almond Breeze Unsweetened Original Almond Milk
- 1/4 cup chia seeds
- 1 tablespoon maple syrup

Chocolate Banana Mousse:
- 1 tablespoon Almond Breeze Unsweetened Original Almond Milk
- 1 large banana
- 1 tablespoon raw cacao powder
- 1 tablespoon almond butter
- 2 tablespoons chia seeds

Smashed Raspberries:

- 1 cup fresh raspberries

Directions.

1. In a bowl, combine Almond Breeze Unsweetened Original Almondmilk, 1/4 cup chia seeds, and maple syrup. Place the mixture in the refrigerator and let it chill for 30 minutes.

2. While the chia mixture is cooling, make the mousse by blending banana, cacao, almond butter, and Almond Breeze Unsweetened Original Almond Milk until smooth and creamy. Pour the mousse into a bowl, mix in 2 tablespoons of chia seeds, and refrigerate until the chia pudding is ready.

3. For the raspberry layer, mash the fresh raspberries in a bowl just before assembling the dessert.

4. To serve, layer the chia pudding, chocolate banana mousse, and mashed raspberries evenly into 3 jars. Enjoy right away or refrigerate for up to 2 days.

Nutritional value
Carbs:51g
Protein:10g
Calories:375
Fat:18g

10.Yogurt Parfait

Prep Time:5 mins
Total Time:5 mins
Serving:2

Ingredients

- 2 cups vanilla yogurt
- 1 cup granola
- 8 blackberries

Directions.

In a large glass, layer 1 cup of yogurt, 1/2 cup of granola, and 4 blackberries; repeat the layers.

Nutritional value
Carbs:68g
Protein:21g
Calories:524
Fat:19g

4.2.Lunches that Sustain and Satisfy

1.Easy Avocado Hummus.

Prep Time:10 mins
Total Time:10 mins
Serving:24

Ingredients
- 1 (15 ounce) can chickpeas, drained
- ¼ cup water

- 2 tablespoons tahini
- 1 tablespoon fresh lime juice, or to taste
- 1 teaspoon sea salt, or to taste
- 1 clove garlic, roughly chopped
- ½ teaspoon ground cumin
- 1 ½ large ripe avocados, pitted and peeled
- 1 bunch spinach leaves
- 2 tablespoons extra-virgin olive oil

Directions.

1.Combine chickpeas, water, tahini, lime juice, salt, garlic, and cumin in a food processor. Blend until smooth for about 2 minutes. Then, add avocados, spinach, and olive oil, and continue blending until creamy, which should take 2 to 3 minutes.

Nutritional value
Carbs:10g
Protein:4g
Calories:75
Fat:4g

2.Black Bean Hummus.

Prep Time:5 mins
Total Time:5 mins
Serving:8

<u>Ingredients</u>

- 1 (15 ounce) can black beans
- 1 clove garlic
- 2 tablespoons lemon juice, or more to taste
- 1½ tablespoons tahini
- ½ teaspoon ground cumin, or more to taste
- ½ teaspoon salt, or more to taste
- ⅛ teaspoon cayenne pepper, or more to taste
- ¼ teaspoon paprika, or as needed
- 10 Greek olives

<u>Directions.</u>

1. Drain the beans, keeping the liquid aside.

2. In a food processor, pulse garlic until finely chopped. Add drained black beans, 2 tablespoons of the reserved bean liquid, lemon juice, tahini, cumin, salt, and cayenne pepper. Blend until smooth, scraping the sides as necessary.

3. Taste and adjust the consistency and flavor by adding more bean liquid, lemon juice, tahini, cumin, salt, or cayenne pepper if desired. Transfer the mixture to a serving bowl and sprinkle with paprika. Garnish with Greek olives on top.

Nutritional value
Carbs:15g
Protein:4g
Calories:85
Fat:5g

3.Seattle Smoked Salmon Dip.

Prep Time:10 mins
Additional Time:1 hr

Total Time:1 hr 10 mins
Serving:20

Ingredients

- 4 ounces flaked smoked salmon, skin and bones removed
- 1 (8 ounce) package cream cheese, softened
- 1 cup shredded white Cheddar cheese, divided
- ½ cup mayonnaise
- 2 tablespoons chopped green onions
- 2 tablespoons milk
- 1 tablespoon lemon juice
- 1 (1 ounce) package McCormick Guacamole Seasoning Mix

Directions.

1. Combine all ingredients in a large bowl until thoroughly mixed. Cover the bowl.

2. Chill in the refrigerator for 1 hour or until you're ready to serve. Optionally, decorate with more green onions before serving.

Nutritional value
Carbs:2g
Protein:3g
Calories:113
Fat:10g

4.Rice Cereal Energy Bars

Prep Time:30 mins
Total Time:30 mins
Serving:24

Ingredients
- ½ cup sesame seeds
- ½ cup sunflower seeds

- 1 pinch salt
- ½ cup chopped dates
- ½ cup raisins
- ½ cup dried apricots
- ½ cup dried cherries
- ½ cup semisweet chocolate chips
- 1 cup rolled oats
- 7 cups crisp rice cereal
- 1 cup corn syrup
- 1 cup white sugar
- 1 ½ cups crunchy peanut butter
- 1 cup powdered milk
- 1 teaspoon vanilla extract
- ½ teaspoon almond extract

Directions.

1. Combine sesame seeds and sunflower seeds in a dry skillet over medium heat. Toast until fragrant, lightly salt, and let cool.

2. Place dates, raisins, apricots, cherries, chocolate chips, and toasted seeds in a food processor. Pulse until chopped finely but not paste-like. Transfer to a large bowl and mix with oats and crisp rice cereal.

3. In a small microwave-safe bowl, combine corn syrup, sugar, and peanut butter. Microwave until bubbly, then stir in powdered milk, vanilla, and almond extract. Pour over the cereal mixture and stir until evenly coated.

4. Press the mixture into a greased 10x15 inch jelly roll pan using wet hands. Cut into squares and let cool completely before removing from the pan.

Nutritional value
Carbs:47g
Protein:8g
Calories:324
Fat:16g

5.Orange-Blueberry-Yogurt Breakfast Parfaits

Prep Time:10 mins
Total Time:10 mins
Serving:2

Ingredients

- ¾ cup vanilla yoghourt
- 1 teaspoon grated orange zest
- 2 large fresh strawberries, sliced
- ¼ cup maple nut granola
- ½ cup fresh blueberries

Directions.

1. Combine yoghourt and orange zest in a bowl.

2. Alternate layers of strawberries, yoghourt mixture, granola, and blueberries in a parfait glass. Repeat layering until all ingredients are used.

Nutritional value
Carbs:55g
Protein:14g
Calories:360
Fat:10g

6.Chickpea Salad with Red Onion and Tomato

Prep Time:10 mins
Total Time:10 mins
Serving:4

Ingredients

- 2 (10.5 ounce) cans chickpeas, drained
- 2 tablespoons red onion, chopped
- 2 cloves garlic, minced
- 1 tomato, chopped
- ½ cup freshly chopped parsley

- 3 tablespoons olive oil
- 1 tablespoon lemon juice
- salt and pepper to taste

Directions.

1.Mix together chickpeas, red onion, garlic, tomato, parsley, olive oil, and lemon juice in a big bowl, and season with salt and pepper as desired.

Nutritional value
Carbs:49g
Protein:15g
Calories:375
Fat:14g

7.Fiery Fish Tacos with Crunchy Corn Salsa.

Prep Time:30 mins
Cook Time:10 mins

Total Time:40 mins
Serving:6

<u>Ingredients</u>

- 2 cups cooked corn kernels
- ½ cup diced red onion
- 1 cup peeled, diced jicama
- ½ cup diced red bell pepper
- 1 cup fresh cilantro leaves, chopped
- 1 lime, juiced and zested
- 2 tablespoons cayenne pepper, or to taste
- 1 tablespoon ground black pepper
- 2 tablespoons salt, or to taste
- 6 (4 ounce) fillets tilapia
- 2 tablespoons olive oil
- 12 corn tortillas, warmed
- 2 tablespoons sour cream, or to taste

<u>Directions.</u>

1. Heat the grill to high temperature.

2. In a medium bowl, combine corn, red onion, jicama, red bell pepper, and cilantro. Mix in lime juice and zest.

3. In a small bowl, blend cayenne pepper, black pepper, and salt.

4. Coat each fillet with olive oil and season with the spice mixture.

5. Place fillets on the grill and cook for 3 minutes on each side. Serve on two corn tortillas per taco, topped with fish, sour cream, and corn salsa.

Nutritional value
Carbs:40g
Protein:29g
Calories:351
Fat:10g

8.Tart Tropical Parfait.

Prep Time:5 mins
Total Time:5 mins

Serving:2

Ingredients

- 1 (5.3 ounce) container low-fat vanilla Greek yoghourt
- ½ cup chopped kiwi
- 2 tablespoons chopped macadamia nuts
- 1 teaspoon agave nectar
- 1 teaspoon chopped fresh mint

Directions.

1."Place 1/3 cup of yoghurt into a 6 to 8-ounce parfait glass or jar. Add half of the kiwi, half of the macadamia nuts, and half of the agave on top of the yoghurt. Repeat these layers with the remaining yoghurt, kiwi, nuts, and agave. Finish by topping the parfait with mint."

Nutritional value

Carbs:37g
Protein:15g
Calories:320
Fat:14g

9.Raspberry Almond Muffins.

Prep Time:20 mins
Cook Time:25 mins
Total Time:45 mins
Serving:6

<u>Ingredients</u>

- 1 cup sliced almonds
- 2 cups all-purpose flour
- ⅔ cup white sugar
- 2 teaspoons baking powder
- ¼ teaspoon baking soda
- 1 teaspoon salt
- ¾ cup warm water
- 2 teaspoons almond extract

- ½ cup butter
- 2 eggs, beaten
- 1 ½ cups frozen raspberries

Directions.

1. Preheat your oven to 375 degrees Fahrenheit (190 degrees Celsius).

2. Spread almonds evenly on a baking sheet and toast in the preheated oven for 5 to 10 minutes until lightly browned.

3. Reduce the oven temperature to 350 degrees Fahrenheit (175 degrees Celsius) and lightly grease a 6-cup jumbo muffin pan.

4. In a medium bowl, combine flour, sugar, 3/4 cup of toasted almonds, baking powder, baking soda, and salt.

5. In another medium bowl, mix together water, almond extract, melted butter, and eggs. Add this mixture to the dry ingredients and blend until combined. Gently fold in raspberries. Spoon the

batter into the prepared muffin pan and sprinkle the tops with the remaining almonds.

6. Bake for 25 minutes at 350 degrees Fahrenheit (175 degrees Celsius) or until a toothpick inserted into the centre of a muffin comes out clean.

Nutritional value
Carbs:78g
Protein:12g
Calories:609
Fat:35g

10.Banana Muffins

Prep Time:10 mins
Cook Time:25 mins
Total Time:35 mins
Serving:12

Ingredients

- 1 ½ cups all-purpose flour
- 1 teaspoon baking powder
- 1 teaspoon baking soda
- ½ teaspoon salt
- 3 large ripe bananas, mashed
- ¾ cup white sugar
- 1 large egg
- ⅓ cup butter, melted

Directions.

1. Preheat your oven to 350 degrees F (175 degrees C). Prepare a 12-cup muffin tin by greasing it or lining the cups with paper liners. In a bowl, sift together flour, baking powder, baking soda, and salt; set aside.

2. In another large bowl, mix together bananas, sugar, egg, and melted butter until thoroughly combined. Gently fold in the flour mixture until the batter is smooth. Spoon the batter into the

prepared muffin cups, filling each about two-thirds full.

3. Bake in the preheated oven for approximately 25 to 30 minutes, or until the tops of the muffins spring back when lightly pressed. Allow them to cool briefly in the muffin tin before transferring them to a wire rack to cool completely.

Nutritional value
Carbs:35g
Protein:5g
Calories:189
Fat:9g

4.3 Dinners that Delight and Heal.

1.Quick Lemon Herb Chicken

Prep Time:5 mins

Cook Time:10 mins
Total Time:15 mins
Serving:2

Ingredients

- 2 (5 ounce) skinless, boneless chicken breast halves
- 1 medium lemon, juiced, divided
- salt and freshly ground black pepper to taste
- 1 tablespoon olive oil
- 1 pinch dried oregano
- 2 sprigs fresh parsley, chopped, for garnish

Directions.

1. Place the chicken in a bowl. Pour half of the lemon juice over the chicken and season with salt.

2. In a medium skillet, heat olive oil over medium-low heat. Place the chicken in the hot oil. Add the remaining lemon juice and oregano, and

season with black pepper. Cook the chicken until it is golden brown and the juices run clear, about 5 to 10 minutes per side. Use an instant-read thermometer to ensure the chicken reaches at least 165 degrees F (74 degrees C) in the thickest part.

3. Garnish the chicken with parsley before serving.

Nutritional value
Carbs:5g
Protein:39g
Calories:275
Fat:11g

2.Grilled Chicken Salad with Seasonal Fruit

Prep Time:15 mins
Cook Time:20 mins
Total Time:35 mins
Serving:6

Ingredients

- 1 pound skinless, boneless chicken breast halves
- ½ cup pecans
- ⅓ cup red wine vinegar
- ½ cup white sugar
- 1 cup vegetable oil
- ½ onion, minced
- 1 teaspoon ground mustard
- 1 teaspoon salt
- ¼ teaspoon ground white pepper
- 2 heads Bibb lettuce - rinsed, dried and torn
- 1 cup sliced fresh strawberries

Directions.

1. Preheat the grill to high and lightly grease the grill grate.

2. Grill the chicken until fully cooked, approximately 8 minutes per side. Once done, let it cool, then slice and set aside.

3. In a dry skillet over medium-high heat, toast the pecans, stirring often, until they become fragrant, about 8 minutes. Remove from heat and set aside.

4. For the dressing: Blend together red wine vinegar, sugar, vegetable oil, onion, mustard, salt, and pepper until smooth.

5. Place lettuce on serving plates. Arrange sliced grilled chicken, strawberries, and pecans on top. Drizzle with the prepared dressing before serving.

Nutritional value
Carbs:23g
Protein:18
Calories:579
Fat:46g

3.Garlic and Rosemary Lemon-Roasted Chicken

Prep Time:30 mins
Cook Time:1 hr 30 mins
Additional Time:10 mins
Total Time:2 hrs 10 mins
Serving:4

<u>Ingredients</u>

- 1 medium lemon
- ½ medium onion
- ½ teaspoon garlic salt
- ½ teaspoon ground sage
- ½ teaspoon ground turmeric
- ½ teaspoon ground thyme
- ½ teaspoon ground basil
- ½ teaspoon ground rosemary
- ½ teaspoon ground black pepper
- 1 (4 pound) whole chicken
- 1 cup arugula
- 6 cloves garlic, peeled and smashed
- 7 tablespoons garlic-infused ghee, divided

- 1 tablespoon butter

Directions.

1. Preheat your oven to 400 degrees F (200 degrees C) and line a baking sheet with foil.

2. Roll the lemon to soften it, then cut it in half lengthwise. Slice one half into quarters and keep the other half aside. Cut the onion into 4 pieces; thinly slice one piece and scatter it on the prepared baking sheet. Set aside the remaining onion pieces.

3. Combine garlic salt, sage, turmeric, basil, rosemary, and pepper in a bowl until mixed well; divide into 2 portions.

4. Rinse the chicken under cold water and pat dry. Remove excess fat and gently separate the skin from the meat. Stuff the chicken cavity with arugula, 4 lemon slices, 3 onion pieces, and garlic cloves. Tie the legs together with kitchen twine. Spread 2

tablespoons of ghee under the skin and another 2 tablespoons over the skin evenly.

5. Mix 2 tablespoons of ghee and butter with one portion of the spice mixture. Microwave for 45 seconds, stir well, and spread it under the chicken skin. Microwave the remaining 1 tablespoon of ghee, brush it over the chicken skin, and sprinkle the remaining spice mixture all over the chicken, patting it gently. Squeeze some of the remaining lemon juice over the chicken and place it breast-side up on the sliced onions on the baking sheet.

6. Bake in the preheated oven for about 1 hour and 30 minutes, basting with pan juices and leftover lemon juice every 30 minutes. Use an instant-read thermometer to ensure the thickest part of the thigh near the bone reaches 165 degrees F (74 degrees C). Remove from the oven, let it rest for 10 minutes before carving, and continue to baste as needed.

Nutritional value
Carbs:8g
Protein:62g
Calories:813
Fat:60g

4.One-Pan Lemon Garlic Chicken and Asparagus.

Prep Time:10 mins
Cook Time:20 mins
Total Time:30 mins
Serving:4

Ingredients

- 6 skinless, boneless chicken thighs (about 2 pounds)
- 1 teaspoon Italian seasoning, or any herb blend
- 1/2 teaspoon paprika

- 1/2 teaspoon garlic powder
- salt and freshly ground black pepper to taste
- 1 tablespoons olive oil
- 1 tablespoon unsalted butter
- 1 cup chicken broth
- 1 pound asparagus, ends trimmed, cut into 1 1/2-inch pieces
- 1 tablespoon minced garlic, or to taste
- 1/2 lemon, juiced
- 4 tablespoons cold unsalted butter
- 1 tablespoon minced fresh parsley
- 1 lemon, sliced (optional)

Directions.

1. Pat dry the chicken thighs and remove any excess fat.

2. In a small bowl, mix together Italian seasoning, paprika, garlic powder, salt, and pepper. Season

both sides of the chicken thighs with this herb mixture.

3. Heat olive oil and 1 tablespoon of butter in a large nonstick skillet over medium heat. Once the oil is hot and butter is melted, add the chicken thighs in a single layer. Cook until browned on both sides, approximately 5 minutes per side. Transfer the chicken to a plate and keep warm.

4. Pour chicken broth into the skillet, scraping up any browned bits, and bring to a boil. Let it boil until the broth reduces by half, about 3 to 5 minutes.

5. Add the asparagus to the skillet and cook, stirring occasionally, until the asparagus turns a deep, bright green colour, usually 3 to 5 minutes.

6. To the asparagus, add fresh garlic and lemon juice. Cook for about 1 minute. Gradually add butter, one tablespoon at a time, stirring until each pat melts completely before adding the next.

7. Return the chicken thighs to the skillet, nestling them into the sauce and asparagus. Sprinkle with

minced parsley and cook until the internal temperature of the chicken reaches 165°F (74°C) when measured with an instant-read thermometer, typically 2 to 3 minutes.

8. Spoon the sauce over the chicken thighs when serving and garnish with lemon slices. Serve the dish warm.

Nutritional value
Carbs:8g
Protein:56g
Calories:661
Fat:48g

5.Lime-Marinated Grilled Salmon.

Prep Time:10 mins
Cook Time:10 mins
Additional Time:1 hr

Total Time:1 hr 20 mins
Serving:4

<u>Ingredients</u>

- ¼ cup fresh lime juice
- 1 tablespoon olive oil
- 2 teaspoons Dijon mustard
- ¼ teaspoon ground ginger
- ¼ teaspoon garlic powder
- ¼ teaspoon cayenne pepper
- ⅛ teaspoon black pepper
- 4 salmon steaks

<u>Directions.</u>

1. Combine lime juice, olive oil, mustard, ginger, garlic, cayenne pepper, and black pepper in a bowl. Transfer to a sealable plastic bag. Add salmon steaks, coat with marinade, remove excess air, and seal. Refrigerate for 1 hour.

2. Preheat an outdoor grill to medium heat and lightly grease the grate. Remove salmon from marinade, shake off excess, and discard remaining marinade.

3. Grill until salmon flakes easily with a fork, about 5 to 10 minutes per side depending on thickness.

Nutritional value
Carbs:2g
Protein:35g
Calories:315
Fat:20g

6.Grilled Rosemary Chicken Breasts.

Prep Time:20 mins
Cook Time:10 mins
Additional Time:30 mins
Total Time:1 hr
Serving:4

Ingredients

- 8 cloves garlic, minced
- 3 tablespoons olive oil
- 2 tablespoons minced fresh rosemary
- 1 ½ tablespoons Dijon mustard
- 1 ½ tablespoons lemon juice
- ¼ teaspoon ground black pepper
- ⅛ teaspoon kosher salt
- 4 boneless, skinless chicken breast halves

Directions.

1. Gather all the necessary ingredients.

2. In a bowl, mix together garlic, oil, rosemary, mustard, lemon juice, pepper, and salt. Set aside 2 tablespoons for later use.

3. Place chicken breasts in a sealable plastic bag. Pour the remaining garlic mixture over the chicken, seal the bag, and massage the marinade into the

chicken. Let it sit at room temperature for 30 minutes.

4. Preheat an outdoor grill to medium-high heat and lightly oil the grate. Remove the chicken from the marinade and shake off any excess. Dispose of the leftover marinade.

5. Grill the chicken for about 4 minutes on one side. Flip the chicken, baste with the reserved marinade, and continue grilling until it is no longer pink in the center and the juices run clear, which should take about 5 more minutes. Ensure the internal temperature reaches at least 165 degrees F (74 degrees C) using an instant-read thermometer. Transfer the grilled chicken to a plate, cover it with foil, and let it rest for at least 2 minutes before serving.

Nutritional value
Carbs:4g
Protein:27g
Calories:238
Fat:14g

7.Honey Grilled Shrimp.

Prep Time:15 mins
Cook Time:5 mins
Additional Time:1 hr
Total Time:1 hr 20 mins
Serving:3

<u>Ingredients</u>

- ½ teaspoon garlic powder
- ¼ tablespoon ground black pepper
- ⅓ cup Worcestershire sauce
- 2 tablespoons dry white wine
- 2 tablespoons Italian-style salad dressing
- 1 pound large shrimp, peeled and deveined with tails attached
- ¼ cup honey
- ¼ cup butter, melted
- 2 tablespoons Worcestershire sauce

- skewers

Directions.

1. Combine garlic powder, black pepper, 1/3 cup Worcestershire sauce, wine, and dressing in a large bowl. Add shrimp and mix well to coat. Cover and refrigerate for 1 hour to marinate.

2. Heat the grill too high. Skewer the shrimp, threading once near the tail and once near the head. Discard the marinade.

3. In a small bowl, mix honey, melted butter, and the remaining 2 tablespoons of Worcestershire sauce. Set aside for basting.

4. Lightly oil the grill grate. Grill the shrimp for 2 to 3 minutes per side until they are opaque. Occasionally baste with the honey-butter sauce while grilling.

Nutritional value
Carbs:33g
Protein:30g

Calories:434g
Fat:20g

8.Lemon and thyme Chicken.

Prep Time:10 mins
Cook Time:10 mins
Additional Time:5 mins
Total Time:25 mins
Serving:4

<u>Ingredients</u>

- 2 tablespoons olive oil
- 1 clove garlic, minced
- 6 sprigs fresh thyme, leaves stripped and chopped
- 1 tablespoon lemon zest
- ¼ cup lemon juice
- salt and pepper to taste
- 1 pound chicken breast tenders

- olive oil-flavoured cooking spray

Directions.

1. Mix olive oil, garlic, thyme, lemon zest, and lemon juice in a large bowl. Season chicken tenders with salt and pepper. Coat chicken with the olive oil mixture and let it marinate for 5 minutes.

2. Spray a non-stick skillet with cooking spray and heat over medium-high. Cook chicken tenders in the skillet until they are golden brown and fully cooked, approximately 4 minutes per side.

Nutritional value
Carbs:3g
Protein:24g
Calories:192
Fat:10g

9.Chicken Stew With Coconut Milk.

Prep Time:15 mins
Cook Time:30 mins
Total Time:45 mins
Serving:6

<u>Ingredients</u>

- 1 pound skinless, boneless chicken breast, cut into bite-sized chunks
- 1 medium yellow onion, chopped or sliced
- 1 cup peeled potatoes, cut in 1-inch chunks
- 1 cup halved baby carrots
- 1 (9 ounce) package frozen baby lima beans
- ¼ (12 ounce) can diced tomatoes
- 1 cup canned coconut milk
- 1 cup fat-free, reduced-sodium chicken broth
- 1 tablespoon cumin
- 1 tablespoon curry powder
- Salt and pepper to taste
- ¼ teaspoon hot sauce (such as Tabasco), or to taste

- Parsley or cilantro for garnish

Directions.

Combine chicken, onion, potatoes, carrots, lima beans, tomatoes, coconut milk, chicken broth, cumin, curry powder, salt, pepper, and hot sauce in a large microwave-safe bowl. Mix well, cover tightly, and microwave on High for 30 to 40 minutes. Sprinkle with parsley or cilantro before serving.

Nutritional value
Carbs:26g
Protein:23g
Calories:265
Fat:11g

4.4 Desserts and Smoothies: Quick Anti-inflammatory Boosts

1.Chocolate Pistachio Cheesecake

Prep Time:1 hr
Cook Time:40 mins
Additional Time:6 hrs
Total Time:7 hrs 40 mins
Serving:8

<u>Ingredients</u>

- 3 ounces chocolate wafer cookies
- ¾ cup raw unsalted pistachios, divided, plus more for garnish
- 2 tablespoons granulated sugar
- 2 tablespoons butter, melted
- 2 (8 ounce) packages reduced-fat cream cheese (Neufchâtel), softened

- 1 avocado, peeled, seeded, and mashed until smooth (1/2 cup)
- 2 cups fat-free plain Greek-style yoghourt
- 2 tablespoons cornstarch
- ¾ cup granulated sugar
- 2 large egg whites
- 1 teaspoon almond extract
- ⅛ teaspoon salt
- ¼ cup whipping cream
- 2 tablespoons powdered sugar
- 1 teaspoon vanilla extract
- 1 (16 ounce) container frozen non dairy low-fat whipped topping, thawed, plus more for garnish

Directions.

1. Preheat your oven to 325 degrees F (165 degrees C). Grease a 9-inch springform pan with cooking spray.

2. Use a food processor to finely grind cookies, 1/4 cup pistachios, and 2 tablespoons of sugar. Leave some texture if desired. Add melted butter and pulse until combined. Press the mixture evenly into the bottom of the prepared pan.

3. To make the pistachio butter, blend the remaining 1/2 cup pistachios in a small food processor until smooth and slightly loose, about 5 minutes. Transfer to a large bowl. Add cream cheese, avocado, 1 cup yoghourt, cornstarch, and 3/4 cup sugar. Use an electric mixer on medium speed until nearly smooth. Add egg whites, almond extract, and a pinch of salt; beat until just combined. Spread this mixture over the crust.

4. Bake until the edges appear set when gently shaken, about 40 minutes. Turn off the oven and let the cheesecake sit inside for 30 minutes. Cool on a wire rack in the pan for 15 minutes. Use a thin metal spatula to loosen the cheesecake from the sides of the pan. Cool completely.

5. For the mousse, beat whipping cream, powdered sugar, vanilla, remaining 1 cup yoghurt, and a pinch of salt in a bowl with an electric mixer until fluffy, about 4 minutes. Spread this mixture over the cooled cheesecake.

6. Top with whipped topping. Cover and chill for at least 4 hours or up to 5 days. To serve, remove from the pan, slice, and garnish with additional whipped topping and pistachios.

Nutritional value
Carbs:81g
Protein:18g
Calories:785
Fat:51g

2.Pumpkin Parfait

Prep Time:15 mins
Additional Time:4 hrs
Total Time:4 hrs 15 mins

Serving:8

<u>Ingredients</u>

- 1 ½ cups graham cracker crumbs
- ¼ cup brown sugar
- ¼ cup melted butter
- 1 (15 ounce) can pure pumpkin
- ½ cup brown sugar
- ¼ teaspoon salt
- ¼ teaspoon ground nutmeg
- ⅛ teaspoon ground cloves
- 1 teaspoon ground cinnamon
- 1 quart vanilla ice cream, softened
- 1 cup whipped cream
- 1 tablespoon confectioners' sugar
- ¼ teaspoon ground cinnamon

<u>Directions.</u>

1. Combine graham cracker crumbs, 1/4 cup of brown sugar, and melted butter in a bowl. Press the

mixture into a 9x9-inch square baking dish to form the crust. In a large bowl, mash the pumpkin and mix in 1/2 cup of brown sugar, salt, nutmeg, cloves, and 1 teaspoon of cinnamon until smooth. Gently fold in softened ice cream. Spread the pumpkin mixture over the graham cracker crust. Freeze until firm, typically 4 to 6 hours, then cut into squares.

2. Lightly blend whipped cream with confectioners' sugar and 1/4 teaspoon of cinnamon in a bowl. Serve each square of the desert with a dollop of the sweetened whipped cream on top.

Nutritional value

Carbs:49g
Protein:6g
Calories:395
Fat:20g

3.Blueberry Bars.

Serving:12

__Ingredients__

- 1 cup all-purpose flour
- 1 ¼ teaspoons baking powder
- ½ cup shortening
- ¾ cup white sugar
- 3 eggs
- ¾ teaspoon almond extract
- ⅓ cup milk
- 1 ½ cups fresh blueberries
- ⅓ cup confectioners' sugar
- 6 tablespoons cream cheese, softened
- 1 teaspoon almond extract

__Directions.__

1. Preheat your oven to 350 degrees Fahrenheit (175 degrees Celsius) and grease a 9-inch square baking dish.

2. For the crust: In a large bowl, combine shortening, sugar, one egg, milk, and almond extract. Add flour and baking powder, mixing well until smooth. Spread the crust evenly in the greased baking dish, then scatter blueberries on top.

3. For the topping: In another bowl, beat two eggs and cream cheese until creamy. Stir in powdered sugar and almond extract until smooth. Spread this mixture over the blueberries.

4. Bake for 55 to 60 minutes, or until the top feels firm to the touch. Allow the baked dish to cool in the pan before cutting into squares.

Nutritional value
Carbs:27g
Protein:6g
Calories:245
Fat:14g

4.Make-Ahead Greek Yogurt Parfait.

Prep Time:10 mins
Total Time:10 mins
Serving:8

Ingredients

- 4 cups nonfat plain Greek yoghourt
- 1 cup granular sucralose sweetener (such as Splenda®)
- 1 ½ teaspoons vanilla extract
- 2 cups granola cereal
- 8 cups frozen mixed fruit, no sugar added

Directions.

1. Mix yoghurt, sweetener, and vanilla extract thoroughly in a large bowl.

2. Distribute 1 cup of frozen fruit into each of 8 plastic cups. Spoon 1/2 cup of the yoghurt mixture over the fruit in each cup. Refrigerate until ready to serve.

3. Before eating, sprinkle 1/4 cup of granola over the yoghurt and fruit in each cup.

Nutritional value
Carbs:63g
Protein:17g
Calories:372
Fat:9g

5.Blackberry Crumble

Prep Time:15 mins
Cook Time:25 mins
Total Time:40 mins
Serving:8

Ingredients

- 4 cups fresh blackberries
- 2 tablespoons white sugar
- 1 cup all-purpose flour

- ½ cup brown sugar
- 6 tablespoons unsalted butter, cubed
- 1 tablespoon ground cinnamon
- ¾ cup chopped walnuts

Directions.

1. Preheat your oven to 375 degrees Fahrenheit (190 degrees Celsius).

2. Spread the blackberries evenly in a large pie dish and sprinkle them with sugar.

3. In a food processor, blend together flour, brown sugar, butter, and cinnamon until well mixed. Crumble this mixture over the berries and sugar in the pie dish. Sprinkle walnuts on top.

4. Bake the dish in your preheated oven until it turns golden and bubbles appear, which should take about 25 to 30 minutes.

Nutritional value
Carbs:39g
Protein:6g
Calories:315

Fat:18g

Chapter 5: Lifestyle Strategies to Complement Your Diet

5.1.The Role of Exercise in Reducing Inflammation.

When we talk about keeping our bodies healthy, exercise often comes up as a go-to solution. It's like a secret ingredient in a chef's kitchen that can transform a simple dish into a gourmet meal. But did you know that exercise isn't just good for your heart and muscles? It's also a powerful tool for fighting inflammation in the body.

How Exercise Reduces Inflammation

Now, let's talk about how exercise comes into play. Imagine exercise as the master spice in your health recipe, reducing the bitterness of inflammation and adding a burst of wellness.

1.Reduces Body Fat: One of the ways exercise helps is by reducing body fat. Excess fat, especially around the abdomen, releases chemicals that promote inflammation. By losing fat through regular physical activity, your body produces fewer of these harmful substances.

2.Boosts Anti-inflammatory Substances: Exercise encourages the production of anti-inflammatory substances in the body. Think of it as stirring in a bit of sweetness to balance out the heat. Regular physical activity increases the levels of cytokines and other molecules that reduce inflammation.

3.Improves Circulation: Good circulation is like a well-mixed batter in a cake. When you exercise, your blood flows more efficiently, delivering oxygen and nutrients to your tissues and removing waste products. This helps keep inflammation under control and promotes healing.

4.Reduces Stress Hormones: Stress can be like too much salt in a dish, making everything worse. Exercise helps reduce the levels of stress hormones like cortisol. High cortisol levels can lead to increased inflammation, so keeping these in check is crucial for a healthy body.

5.Enhances Immune Function: Regular exercise strengthens your immune system, making it more effective at fighting off infections and illnesses. This means your body is better prepared to handle the stresses that can trigger inflammation.

Types of Exercise That Help

Not all exercise is created equal when it comes to fighting inflammation. Here are some types of activities that are particularly effective:

1.Aerobic Exercise: Activities like walking, jogging, swimming, and cycling are great for getting your heart rate up. They improve cardiovascular health and help reduce inflammation throughout the body.

2.Strength Training: Lifting weights or doing body-weight exercises like push-ups and squats builds muscle. More muscle means a higher metabolism and less fat, which contributes to lower inflammation levels.

3.Flexibility and Balance Exercises: Yoga and tai chi are excellent for reducing stress and improving circulation. These practices also promote mindfulness and relaxation, helping to lower stress hormones.

4.Moderate to Vigorous Activities: Aim for a mix of moderate and vigorous activities. Even gardening or a brisk walk can make a big difference. The key is consistency and finding something you enjoy, so you stick with it.

Tips for Getting Started

If you're new to exercise, don't worry. You don't have to run a marathon tomorrow. Start small and gradually increase your activity level. Here are a few tips to get you moving:

Set Realistic Goals: Begin with simple, achievable goals. Maybe it's a 10-minute walk each day or a few minutes of stretching in the morning.

Find Your Passion: Choose activities that you enjoy. Whether it's dancing, hiking, or playing a sport, make it fun.

Stay Consistent: Consistency is key. Aim for at least 30 minutes of moderate exercise most days of the week.

Listen to Your Body: Pay attention to how your body feels. Rest when you need to, and don't push too hard too fast.

Get Support: Find a friend or join a class to keep you motivated. Having a support system can make a big difference.

5.2.Stress Management Techniques: Meditation, Yoga, and More

Stress is more than just a mental or emotional state. It affects our entire body, and chronic stress can lead to inflammation. This inflammation can contribute to serious health issues like heart disease, arthritis, and even some cancers. Thankfully, there are techniques that can help manage stress and, in turn, reduce inflammation. Let's explore how meditation, yoga, and a few other strategies can play a crucial role in stress relief and anti-inflammatory benefits.

Meditation: A Moment of Peace

Meditation is like a reset button for your mind. It's about taking a few minutes each day to focus and breathe deeply. This simple act helps calm the nervous system, reducing the levels of stress hormones like cortisol. High cortisol levels are linked to inflammation, so by lowering them, meditation helps keep inflammation in check.

Think of meditation as giving your brain a mini-vacation. When you close your eyes and concentrate on your breath or a soothing word, you give your brain a break from the constant bombardment of daily stress. This not only improves mental clarity but also has a physical impact. Studies show that regular meditation can decrease inflammatory markers in the body, making it a powerful tool for overall health.

Yoga: Moving with Purpose

Yoga combines physical postures, breathing exercises, and meditation. It's like a three-in-one approach to stress management and health. When you practise yoga, you're not just stretching your muscles; you're also learning to breathe more deeply and focus your mind.

The physical poses in yoga help increase flexibility and strength, but they also have a deeper impact. Moving and holding these poses can stimulate the vagus nerve, which plays a significant role in the body's ability to relax and lower inflammation. The deep breathing associated with yoga promotes relaxation and reduces stress, further aiding in lowering inflammation.

Moreover, yoga teaches mindfulness, which is the practice of being present in the moment without judgement. This mindfulness can help break the cycle of stress and inflammation by keeping your thoughts from racing and allowing you to focus on the now.

Breathing Techniques: Calm in Every Breath

Breathing might seem like a simple, automatic process, but the way you breathe can significantly affect your stress levels and inflammation. Controlled breathing techniques, like diaphragmatic breathing or the 4-7-8 method, can activate the body's relaxation response.

When you breathe deeply and slowly, it sends a signal to your brain that everything is okay. This signal helps to lower your heart rate and blood pressure, reducing stress and its inflammatory impact. Practising these techniques regularly can help keep your body in a state of calm, even in stressful situations.

Tai Chi: Gentle Flow

Tai Chi is another excellent stress-relief technique. It's a form of exercise that involves slow, deliberate movements and deep breathing. Often described as "meditation in motion," Tai Chi is gentle on the body and suitable for all fitness levels.

The slow, flowing movements of Tai Chi help improve balance, flexibility, and strength. They also promote relaxation and reduce stress, which can lower inflammation. By focusing on the flow of movement and the breath, Tai Chi helps clear the mind and relax the body, making it an effective way to combat stress and inflammation.

Adequate Sleep: The Healing Time

Sleep is essential for health and well-being. During sleep, your body repairs itself and reduces inflammation. Chronic lack of sleep increases stress hormones and inflammatory markers, making it crucial to get enough rest each night.

Practising good sleep hygiene can improve the quality of your sleep. This includes maintaining a regular sleep schedule, creating a restful environment, and avoiding stimulants like caffeine close to bedtime. Quality sleep helps keep your stress and inflammation in check.

Nutrition: Feeding Your Calm

What you eat can also affect your stress levels and inflammation. A diet rich in fruits, vegetables, whole grains, and healthy fats can help reduce inflammation. Foods like leafy greens, berries, nuts, and fatty fish are known for their anti-inflammatory properties.

Avoiding processed foods, sugar, and excessive alcohol can also help manage inflammation. Staying hydrated and eating balanced meals at regular intervals can keep your energy levels steady and reduce stress.

5.3 Sleep: The Restorative Power for Reducing Inflammation.

When we think about staying healthy, most of us focus on what we eat or how often we exercise. But there's another crucial element that often gets overlooked: sleep. Just like a seasoned chef knows the secret to a perfect dish, a good night's sleep is key to maintaining our body's balance. Let's explore how sleep helps reduce inflammation and why it's essential for our well-being.

The Role of Sleep in Reducing Inflammation

Sleep is not just a time for rest; it's when your body goes into repair mode. During sleep, your body releases proteins called cytokines. Some cytokines promote sleep, while others help fight infection, stress, and inflammation. Without enough sleep, your body makes fewer protective cytokines and more of the inflammatory ones. This imbalance can increase inflammation and lower your body's defences.

A good analogy is to think of sleep as a reset button. Just like how we recharge our phones overnight, sleep recharges our body. It helps clear out the "junk" accumulated during the day, including inflammatory markers. Without adequate sleep, these markers can build up, leading to higher levels of inflammation.

How Lack of Sleep Affects Inflammation

Consider a time when you didn't get enough sleep. Maybe you felt tired, irritable, or even had a headache. Lack of sleep does more than just make us feel lousy; it affects our body on a deeper level. Research shows that even one night of poor sleep can increase inflammation. If you regularly skimp on sleep, the effects can be even more significant.

Chronic sleep deprivation is like letting a pot simmer for too long. Over time, the heat builds up, and things start to boil over. Similarly, without enough sleep, inflammation can build up in your body, increasing the risk of chronic diseases.

Tips for Better Sleep to Reduce Inflammation

Now that we understand the importance of sleep, let's look at some practical tips to improve sleep quality and reduce inflammation.

1.Stick to a Sleep Schedule: Go to bed and wake up at the same time every day, even on weekends. Consistency helps regulate your body's internal clock, making it easier to fall asleep and wake up.

2.Create a Relaxing Bedtime Routine: Just as a chef prepares ingredients before cooking, preparing for sleep is crucial. Wind down with calming activities like reading, listening to soothing music, or taking a warm bath.

3.Watch What You Eat and Drink: Avoid heavy meals, caffeine, and alcohol close to bedtime. These can disrupt your sleep cycle and make it harder to get restorative sleep.

4.Keep Your Sleep Environment Comfortable: Your bedroom should be cool, quiet, and dark. Consider investing in a good mattress and pillows, and minimise noise and light.

5.Limit Screen Time Before Bed:

The blue light from screens can interfere with your sleep. Try to turn off electronic devices at least an hour before bedtime.

6.Stay Active, But Not Too Late: Regular physical activity helps you fall asleep faster and enjoy deeper sleep. However, try to avoid vigorous exercise close to bedtime as it can keep you awake.

The Bigger Picture

Sleep is a vital part of our health, just like a balanced diet and regular exercise. It's when our body takes the time to repair, regenerate, and reset. By prioritising good sleep, we can keep inflammation at bay and protect our long-term health.

So, think of your bed as your body's kitchen – a place where the essential ingredients for health and well-being come together. With the right amount of sleep, you can wake up feeling refreshed, recharged, and ready to take on whatever comes your way.

Remember, the recipe for reducing inflammation isn't just about what's on your plate or how much you move. It's also about how well you sleep. So, tuck yourself in and give your body the rest it needs. You'll be cooking up a healthier, happier you in no time.

5.4.Detoxifying Your Environment: Reducing Toxins at Home

Kitchen Clean-Up

The kitchen is often the heart of the home, where we prepare nutritious meals. To reduce toxins here, start by examining the materials you use for cooking and storing food.

1.Choose Safe Cookware: Non-stick pans can release harmful chemicals when heated. Opt for alternatives like stainless steel, cast iron, or ceramic. These materials not only cook your food evenly but also avoid leaching toxins.

2.Avoid Plastic: Plastics can contain chemicals like BPA and phthalates, which may contribute to inflammation. Use glass or stainless-steel containers for food storage. For drinking, switch to reusable glass or stainless-steel bottles.

3.Buy Organic: Pesticides in non-organic produce can increase your toxin load. Whenever possible, choose organic fruits and vegetables. Washing your produce thoroughly, even if it's organic, can help remove residues.

4.Filter Your Water: Tap water can contain chlorine, lead, and other contaminants. A good water filter can reduce these toxins. Consider a filter that removes a broad range of contaminants to ensure your water is clean.

Air Quality

Breathing clean air is crucial for reducing inflammation and supporting overall health. Here's how to improve your indoor air quality:

1.Ventilate: Open your windows regularly to allow fresh air to circulate. Use exhaust fans when cooking to reduce indoor air pollutants.

2.Use Air Purifiers: Invest in a high-quality air purifier to remove pollutants like dust, pet dander, and volatile organic compounds (VOCs). Look for purifiers with HEPA filters, which are effective at capturing small particles.

3.Houseplants: Some plants, like spider plants and peace lilies, can help purify the air. They absorb toxins and release oxygen, making your home healthier and more pleasant.

4.Avoid Synthetic Fragrances: Air fresheners, scented candles, and other fragranced products often contain chemicals that can irritate your respiratory system. Opt for natural alternatives, such as essential oils, or simply use good ventilation to keep your home smelling fresh.

Cleaning Products

Many conventional cleaning products contain harsh chemicals that can contribute to inflammation. Switch to safer, natural options:

1.Read Labels: Choose products labelled as non-toxic, biodegradable, or free from harsh chemicals. Ingredients like vinegar, baking soda, and castile soap can be effective and safe for cleaning.

2.DIY Cleaners: Make your own cleaning solutions using simple ingredients. For example, a mix of vinegar and water can clean glass and surfaces, while baking soda works well for scrubbing.

3.Avoid Aerosols: Aerosol sprays can release harmful particles into the air. Use pump sprays or wipe-on products instead.

Personal Care

The products you use on your body can be a significant source of toxins. Reduce your exposure with these tips:

1.Check Ingredients: Look for personal care products free of parabens, sulphates, and synthetic fragrances. These chemicals can disrupt hormones and cause skin irritation.

2.Go Natural: Use products with natural ingredients. For instance, coconut oil can be an excellent moisturiser, and essential oils can be used as natural perfumes.

3.Simplify Your Routine: Reduce the number of products you use daily. The fewer products you apply to your skin and hair, the fewer toxins you introduce to your body.

Reducing Electromagnetic Fields (EMFs)

We are surrounded by devices that emit EMFs, which can impact our health over time. Here's how to minimise exposure:

1.Limit Device Use: Turn off Wi-Fi routers at night and keep electronic devices away from your bedroom. This reduces your exposure while you sleep.

2.Use Wired Connections: When possible, use wired connections for your internet and phone to reduce EMF exposure from wireless signals.

3.Keep Devices at a Distance: Avoid keeping your phone in your pocket or using your laptop directly on your lap. Use headphones or speaker mode to keep devices away from your head when making calls.

Creating a Calm Space

Lastly, your home should be a sanctuary that supports relaxation and well-being. A calm environment helps reduce stress, a significant contributor to inflammation.

1.Declutter: A tidy space can reduce stress and improve your mood. Keep your home organised and free from unnecessary items.

2.Use Natural Light: Natural light can enhance your mood and regulate your sleep patterns. Open your curtains during the day and spend time outside when you can.

3.Incorporate Calm Colours: Use soothing colours like blues and greens in your decor to create a relaxing atmosphere.

By making these changes, you can significantly reduce toxins in your home, support your body's natural anti-inflammatory processes, and create a healthier living environment. Small steps can lead to big improvements in how you feel and function every day.

5.5 Supplements and Natural Remedies: Enhancing Your Diet

1. Omega-3 Fatty Acids

Omega-3 fatty acids are superstar nutrients when it comes to fighting inflammation. Found in fatty fish like salmon, mackerel, and sardines, these healthy fats help reduce the production of inflammatory molecules in the body. If you're not a fan of fish, flaxseeds, chia seeds, and walnuts are excellent plant-based sources.

For those who struggle to get enough omega-3s through diet alone, fish oil supplements can be a great option. Look for high-quality, purified fish oil supplements that provide at least 1,000 milligrams of EPA and DHA, the active forms of omega-3s.

2. Turmeric and Curcumin

Turmeric, a golden spice commonly used in Indian cuisine, is well-known for its anti-inflammatory properties. The magic lies in curcumin, the active compound in turmeric. Curcumin has been extensively studied for its ability to combat inflammation and is often recommended for conditions like arthritis.

To get the most out of turmeric, pair it with black pepper. The piperine in black pepper enhances the absorption of curcumin. You can add turmeric to your meals, or take it as a supplement. Look for curcumin supplements that contain piperine or are labelled as "enhanced absorption."

3. Ginger

Ginger is another culinary favourite that packs a punch against inflammation. Known for its spicy kick, ginger has compounds called gingerols and shogaols that help reduce inflammation and pain. Fresh ginger can be grated into teas, soups, and stir-fries, adding both flavour and health benefits.

Ginger supplements are also available and can be particularly useful for those dealing with chronic pain or inflammatory conditions. Just be sure to choose a supplement with a high concentration of ginger extract.

4. Green Tea

Green tea is a soothing drink that offers more than just comfort. It contains a compound called EGCG (epigallocatechin gallate) which has powerful anti-inflammatory effects. Drinking a few cups of green tea each day can help reduce inflammation and provide other health benefits like improved brain function and fat loss.

For those who prefer a stronger dose, green tea extract supplements are available. These can be an easy way to reap the benefits without having to drink multiple cups of tea each day.

5. Probiotics

Gut health is closely linked to inflammation. A healthy gut can help keep inflammation in check, while an unhealthy gut can contribute to it. Probiotics are beneficial bacteria that support gut health. They can be found in fermented foods like yoghurt, kefir, sauerkraut, and kimchi.

Probiotic supplements are a convenient way to ensure you're getting enough of these good bacteria. Look for a broad-spectrum probiotic that contains a variety of strains and has a high colony-forming unit (CFU) count.

6. Antioxidant-Rich Foods

Antioxidants help protect our cells from damage that can trigger inflammation. Berries, dark leafy greens, nuts, and seeds are packed with these protective compounds. Incorporating a variety of these foods into your daily diet can help reduce inflammation and support overall health.

Supplements like vitamin C, vitamin E, and selenium can also boost your antioxidant intake.

These can be particularly beneficial if your diet lacks sufficient fruits and vegetables.

7. Garlic

Garlic is more than just a flavour booster. It contains sulphur compounds that have strong anti-inflammatory effects. Adding fresh garlic to your meals not only enhances the taste but also provides these health benefits.

For those who prefer not to deal with garlic breath, garlic supplements are available. Aged garlic extract is a popular choice because it's odourless and retains the anti-inflammatory properties of fresh garlic.

Incorporating Supplements and Remedies

To get the most out of these supplements and natural remedies, consistency is key. Make them a regular part of your diet rather than occasional additions. Start with one or two supplements and monitor how your body responds. Remember, supplements are most effective when combined with a balanced diet rich in whole, unprocessed foods.

Inflammation can be a silent but powerful foe. By choosing the right foods and supplements, you can arm yourself with the tools to fight it and enhance your health. Whether it's a splash of turmeric in your morning smoothie, a daily fish oil capsule, or a soothing cup of green tea, these small changes can make a big difference in your wellness journey.

Chapter 6: Monitoring and Sustaining an Anti-inflammatory Lifestyle

6.1.Tracking Progress: Tools and Techniques

Eating to fight inflammation can transform your health, but staying on track can be challenging. Like preparing a complex dish, it's about blending the right ingredients, techniques, and timing. Whether you're just starting or refining your approach, knowing how to track your progress can make all the difference. Here's a simple guide to keep you cooking up success in your anti-inflammatory journey.

Understand Your Goals

Before we dive into the practical tools and techniques, it's crucial to set clear, realistic goals. Are you aiming to reduce chronic pain, manage an autoimmune condition, or improve overall well-being? Identifying your primary objectives will help you measure your progress accurately.

Keep a Food Diary

One of the most straightforward and effective tools is a food diary. Write down everything you eat and drink each day. It's like keeping a log of ingredients in your favorite recipe. Note the time of day, portion sizes, and any symptoms you experience. This helps you spot patterns and triggers. Are you noticing more joint pain after consuming certain foods? Does your energy spike or drop at specific times? This data is invaluable in understanding how your body responds to different foods.

Use Apps and Online Tools

In today's digital age, there are numerous apps designed to help track dietary habits. Apps like MyFitnessPal or Cronometer allow you to log your meals and monitor your nutrient intake. They often include features for tracking calories, macros, and even inflammation markers. These apps can provide detailed insights into your diet and help ensure you're getting enough anti-inflammatory nutrients, like omega-3 fatty acids and antioxidants.

Monitor Symptoms and Health Metrics

Besides tracking what you eat, it's essential to monitor your health metrics and symptoms. Regularly check your weight, blood pressure, and other relevant health indicators. Keeping a journal of symptoms like pain levels, fatigue, and mood can show how closely your diet and well-being are linked. For a more detailed picture, consider using wearable devices like fitness trackers that can monitor sleep, activity levels, and heart rate.

Regular Medical Check-Ups

Regular check-ups with your healthcare provider are vital. Blood tests can measure inflammation levels in your body, such as C-reactive protein (CRP) and erythrocyte sedimentation rate (ESR). Your doctor can also help track changes in conditions like arthritis or digestive disorders. This professional insight complements your personal tracking efforts and helps tailor your anti-inflammatory strategy effectively.

Set Short-Term Milestones

Like perfecting a new dish, reaching your health goals happens step by step. Set small, achievable milestones. For example, aim to reduce soda intake by half within a month or incorporate two servings of leafy greens into your daily meals. Celebrate these small victories; they keep you motivated and make the long-term goals seem more attainable.

Educate Yourself

Understanding the "why" behind anti-inflammatory foods can keep you motivated.

Educate yourself about the benefits of ingredients like turmeric, ginger, and leafy greens. Learn how omega-3 fatty acids found in fish can lower inflammation or how antioxidants in berries protect your cells. The more you know, the more empowered you'll feel to make the right choices.

Seek Support

Going it alone can be tough. Join a support group, either online or in your community, where you can share experiences and tips with others. Sometimes, just knowing others are on the same path can be a huge motivator. Consider working with a dietitian or nutrition coach who can provide personalised advice and keep you accountable.

Adjust and Adapt

Flexibility is key. As you track your progress, you might find that some foods you thought were beneficial don't suit you, or you might discover new favourites. Be open to adjusting your plan. Just like tweaking a recipe to perfect a dish, fine-tuning your diet based on what you learn can lead to better results.

Reflect and Reward Yourself

Finally, take time to reflect on your progress regularly. Look back at your food diary, health metrics, and symptoms journal to see how far you've come. Reward yourself for your efforts, whether it's with a relaxing day off, a new kitchen gadget, or simply enjoying a favourite anti-inflammatory meal.

6.2.Adjusting Your Plan: Responding to Changes in Your Body

When you decide to start an anti-inflammatory diet, it's like getting to know your body all over again. As a seasoned chef, I've learned that food is not just about taste; it's also about how it makes you feel. The same applies to an anti-inflammatory diet. You need to pay close attention to your body and adjust your plan as necessary.

Starting the Diet

When you start eating anti-inflammatory foods, you might notice some changes quickly. You could feel more energetic, and your mood might improve. This is your body's way of telling you that it likes the changes you're making.

Start by incorporating foods like fresh fruits and vegetables, whole grains, lean proteins, and healthy fats like olive oil and avocados. These foods are packed with nutrients and help reduce inflammation naturally. Avoid processed foods, sugar, and trans fats, which can trigger inflammation.

Listening to Your Body

As you continue with your diet, keep an eye on how your body responds. Everyone is different, and what works for one person might not work for another. Pay attention to any signs of discomfort or changes in your health.

For example, you might notice that certain foods cause bloating or digestive issues. This could be your body's way of signalling that those foods aren't right for you. On the other hand, if you feel more energetic after eating certain meals, take note of what you ate.

Adjusting Your Diet

If you experience any adverse reactions, don't be afraid to make adjustments. For instance, if dairy or gluten causes discomfort, consider reducing or eliminating these from your diet. Substitute with alternatives like almond milk or gluten-free grains.

It's also important to stay hydrated. Drinking plenty of water can help your body flush out toxins and reduce inflammation. Herbal teas and broths can also be soothing and beneficial.

Keeping It Balanced

Balance is key in an anti-inflammatory diet. Make sure you're getting a variety of nutrients. Include different types of vegetables, proteins, and healthy fats in your meals. This not only helps in fighting inflammation but also ensures you enjoy your meals.

Meal Planning Tips

Planning your meals can make it easier to stick to an anti-inflammatory diet. Here are a few tips to help you:

Prep Ahead: Spend some time each week chopping vegetables, cooking grains, and preparing proteins. This makes it easier to assemble meals quickly.

Keep It Simple: You don't need elaborate recipes. Simple dishes like grilled chicken with roasted vegetables or a salad with a variety of greens and a drizzle of olive oil can be delicious and satisfying.

Experiment with Spices: Many spices, like turmeric and ginger, have anti-inflammatory properties. Experiment with adding these to your meals for both flavour and health benefits.

Seeking Professional Guidance

While it's great to take charge of your diet, consulting a healthcare professional or a dietitian can provide you with tailored advice. They can help you understand which foods are best for your specific needs and ensure that you're not missing out on essential nutrients.

Staying Patient

Adjusting to a new way of eating takes time. Be patient with yourself and give your body time to adapt. It might take a few weeks or even months to notice significant changes, but it's worth it.

Remember, an anti-inflammatory diet is not just about avoiding certain foods; it's about embracing a healthier way of eating that makes you feel good from the inside out.

Reflect and Adjust

Every few weeks, take some time to reflect on how you feel. Are you experiencing less pain or discomfort? Do you have more energy? Use this feedback to make any necessary adjustments to your diet.

In the kitchen, we often tweak recipes to get the perfect flavour. Similarly, you might need to tweak your diet to get the best results for your health.

6.3.Staying Motivated: Tips and Tricks

I understand the power of food—not just in creating delicious meals but also in nurturing our bodies and fighting inflammation. Adopting an anti-inflammatory diet can feel overwhelming at first, but with the right mindset and a few practical strategies, you can stay motivated and make this lifestyle enjoyable and sustainable.

Understand the Why Behind Your Choice

First and foremost, it's essential to grasp why you're choosing an anti-inflammatory diet. This way of eating isn't just a trend; it has profound benefits for your health. Chronic inflammation is linked to numerous health issues, from arthritis to heart disease. By focusing on anti-inflammatory foods, you're not just following a diet—you're investing in your long-term well-being.

Start with Small Changes

Don't feel like you have to overhaul your entire eating plan overnight. Start small. Swap out one inflammatory food for a healthier option each week. For instance, replace sugary snacks with fresh fruits or choose whole grains over refined ones. These small, manageable changes can build momentum and make the transition smoother.

Stock Up on Staples

Keeping your kitchen well-stocked with anti-inflammatory staples is key. Think colourful fruits and vegetables, fatty fish like salmon, nuts, seeds, olive oil, and whole grains. Having these ingredients readily available makes it easier to prepare healthy meals without feeling restricted.

Plan and Prep Ahead

Life gets busy, and it's easy to reach for convenient, less healthy options when you're short on time. Prevent this by planning and prepping your meals in advance. Spend a couple of hours on the weekend chopping vegetables, cooking grains, and portioning out snacks. This way, you have nutritious meals ready to go throughout the week, reducing the temptation to stray from your diet.

Experiment with New Recipes

An anti-inflammatory diet doesn't have to be boring. Explore new recipes that excite your palate and incorporate a variety of flavours. Try dishes from different cuisines that use herbs and spices known for their anti-inflammatory properties, like turmeric, ginger, and garlic. Cooking should be a delightful experience, and discovering new favourites can keep your motivation high.

Set Realistic Goals

Setting attainable goals is crucial for staying motivated. Rather than aiming for perfection, focus on gradual improvement. Celebrate small victories, whether it's trying a new anti-inflammatory recipe or sticking to your diet for a week straight. These milestones will keep you encouraged and eager to continue.

Find a Support System

Surround yourself with people who support your choices. Whether it's family, friends, or an online community, having a support system can provide encouragement and accountability. Share your progress, exchange recipes, and discuss challenges. Knowing you're not alone on this path can be incredibly motivating.

Listen to Your Body

Pay attention to how your body responds to different foods. Notice the changes in your energy levels, mood, and overall well-being. Positive feedback from your body can be a powerful motivator. When you feel the benefits of eating anti-inflammatory foods, you'll be more inclined to stick with it.

Allow for Flexibility

Remember, it's okay to indulge occasionally. An anti-inflammatory diet is about balance, not restriction. Allow yourself some flexibility to enjoy your favourite treats in moderation. This prevents feelings of deprivation and makes it easier to maintain your diet in the long run.

Keep Learning

Stay informed about the latest research and tips on anti-inflammatory eating. Read books, follow credible blogs, and watch documentaries. The more you learn, the more inspired you'll be to continue making healthy choices.

Reflect on Your Progress

Take time to reflect on how far you've come. Whether you've noticed physical improvements, discovered new recipes, or simply feel better about your food choices, acknowledging your progress reinforces your motivation.

Chapter 7: Future Trends and Innovations in Anti-inflammatory Living

7.1 The Latest Research: What Science Says About Inflammation

The Hidden Dangers of Chronic Inflammation

Recent studies have revealed that chronic inflammation plays a significant role in many serious health conditions. Researchers have found links between chronic inflammation and diseases like heart disease, diabetes, cancer, and even Alzheimer's disease. In these cases, inflammation doesn't just act as a symptom but is a part of the disease process itself.

For example, in heart disease, chronic inflammation can damage the lining of the arteries. This damage leads to the buildup of plaques, which can block blood flow and potentially cause heart attacks or strokes. In diabetes, chronic inflammation can interfere with insulin signalling, making it harder for the body to regulate blood sugar levels. And in the brain, chronic inflammation is believed to contribute to the development and progression of Alzheimer's disease by damaging neurons and disrupting communication between them.

New Frontiers in Inflammation Research

Scientists are continuously exploring new ways to manage and treat inflammation. One promising area is the study of natural compounds found in foods. For instance, curcumin, a compound in turmeric, and resveratrol, found in red wine, have been shown to have anti-inflammatory properties. Research is ongoing to understand how these compounds work and how they can be used effectively in treatments.

Another exciting development is in the field of personalised medicine. By understanding an individual's genetic makeup and unique inflammatory responses, doctors may be able to tailor treatments more precisely. This approach could lead to better management of inflammatory diseases and more effective prevention strategies.

7.2.Innovations in Anti-inflammatory Foods and Supplements.

Turmeric and Curcumin

Turmeric, a spice commonly used in Indian cuisine, has been celebrated for its anti-inflammatory properties. The active ingredient in turmeric, curcumin, is the main reason behind these benefits. Recent advancements have focused on making curcumin more bioavailable, meaning it's easier for our bodies to absorb. New formulations, like curcumin nanoparticles and curcumin combined with piperine (from black pepper), significantly increase its absorption, maximising its potential to reduce inflammation.

Omega-3 Fatty Acids

Omega-3 fatty acids, found in fish oil, flaxseeds, and walnuts, are well-known for their ability to combat inflammation. These fats reduce the production of inflammatory molecules in the body. Innovations in omega-3 supplements include higher concentrations of EPA and DHA (the active components) and the development of algae-based omega-3, offering a plant-based alternative that's especially appealing to vegetarians and vegans.

Cannabidiol (CBD)

CBD, derived from the cannabis plant, is gaining popularity for its anti-inflammatory effects without the psychoactive properties of THC. Researchers are exploring various delivery methods, such as oils, capsules, and topical creams, to see which is most effective for reducing inflammation. New products often combine CBD with other anti-inflammatory compounds, enhancing their overall effectiveness.

Polyphenols

Polyphenols are antioxidants found in many fruits and vegetables. They play a significant role in fighting inflammation and protecting cells from damage. Resveratrol, found in grapes and red wine, and quercetin, found in apples and onions, are two powerful polyphenols. Recent studies suggest that combining different polyphenols can create a synergistic effect, boosting their anti-inflammatory power more than when used alone.

Fermented Foods and Probiotics

The gut plays a crucial role in regulating inflammation throughout the body. Fermented foods like yoghourt, kimchi, and sauerkraut are rich in probiotics—beneficial bacteria that help maintain a healthy gut microbiome. Innovations in this area include new strains of probiotics specifically designed to reduce inflammation and the development of prebiotics, which are fibres that feed these beneficial bacteria, enhancing their effectiveness.

Ginger

Ginger has long been used in traditional medicine for its anti-inflammatory properties. It contains compounds like gingerol and shogaol, which help reduce inflammation and pain. New ginger supplements often concentrate these active compounds and are formulated to improve absorption and effectiveness, making it easier to get significant anti-inflammatory benefits from smaller doses.

Tart Cherry Juice

Tart cherry juice is becoming a popular natural remedy for inflammation and muscle recovery. It's rich in anthocyanins, which have potent anti-inflammatory effects. Recent innovations include concentrated tart cherry supplements and freeze-dried powders, making it more convenient to incorporate these benefits into daily life without the need to drink large volumes of juice.

Green Tea Extract

Green tea is another powerful anti-inflammatory food, primarily due to its high content of catechins, particularly EGCG (epigallocatechin gallate). Advances in green tea extract supplements have focused on increasing the concentration of EGCG and ensuring it remains stable and bioavailable in the body, providing a strong anti-inflammatory effect even in small amounts.

Collagen

Collagen supplements, often sourced from animals or fish, are increasingly recognized for their role in supporting joint health and reducing inflammation. New collagen formulations include hydrolyzed collagen, which is easier for the body to absorb, and multi-collagen blends that combine different types of collagen for broader benefits.

Adaptogens

Adaptogens like ashwagandha, rhodiola, and holy basil help the body adapt to stress, which is a major trigger for inflammation. Recent innovations in adaptogen supplements focus on combining these herbs with other anti-inflammatory compounds, creating potent blends that not only reduce inflammation but also support overall well-being.

7.3 Tech and Tools: Apps and Gadgets for Health Monitoring.

Wearable Health Monitors

1.Fitness Trackers:

Modern fitness trackers, like Fitbit and Garmin, do more than count steps. They monitor heart rate, sleep patterns, and activity levels. Elevated heart rates and poor sleep quality can be signs of increased inflammation. These devices provide data that can be crucial for identifying inflammation early and taking proactive steps to address it.

2.Smartwatches:

Apple Watch and Samsung Galaxy Watch go beyond fitness tracking. They can monitor heart health, oxygen levels, and even perform ECGs. Abnormal readings can indicate underlying inflammation or other health issues. These watches allow continuous monitoring, providing a comprehensive overview of your health in real time.

3.Continuous Glucose Monitors (CGMs):

For those with diabetes or pre-diabetes, CGMs like the Dexcom G6 offer a window into how blood sugar levels fluctuate throughout the day. Spikes in blood sugar can lead to inflammation. By keeping blood sugar stable, CGMs help reduce inflammatory responses in the body.

Mobile Apps for Inflammation Monitoring

1.MyFitnessPal:

Nutrition plays a significant role in managing inflammation. MyFitnessPal helps users track their food intake, focusing on nutrients that can reduce inflammation. It also allows you to monitor how your diet affects your energy levels and overall health.

2.Headspace:

Stress is a known trigger for inflammation. Headspace provides guided meditation and mindfulness exercises to help reduce stress. Regular use can lower stress hormones, leading to reduced inflammation and better mental health.

3.Sleep Cycle:

Quality sleep is crucial for keeping inflammation at bay. Sleep Cycle tracks your sleep patterns and helps you understand how lifestyle factors affect your rest. Better sleep translates to lower levels of inflammatory markers in the body.

4.PainScale:

Chronic pain is often associated with inflammation. PainScale allows users to track their pain levels and identify triggers. This can help in managing conditions like arthritis and fibromyalgia, providing insights into how different treatments and lifestyle changes impact inflammation.

Advanced Health Gadgets

1.Body Composition Scales:

Devices like the Withings Body+ provide detailed insights into your body composition. Understanding your muscle mass, fat percentage, and visceral fat levels can help in managing inflammation. Excess visceral fat is linked to higher levels of inflammation, so keeping it in check is crucial.

2.Thermographic Cameras:

These specialized cameras can detect heat patterns in the body. Areas of inflammation often show higher temperatures. Though more commonly used in clinical settings, consumer versions are becoming available, offering another way to monitor inflammation.

3.Heart Rate Variability (HRV) Monitors:

HRV is a measure of the variation in time between each heartbeat. Lower HRV is associated with higher stress and inflammation. Devices like Oura Ring or Elite HRV provide insights into your HRV, helping you understand how your body responds to stress and recovery.

Integrating Technology into Daily Life

To effectively use these tools, it's essential to integrate them into your daily routine. Start by selecting a few devices or apps that fit your lifestyle and health needs. Use fitness trackers and smartwatches to gather continuous data on your activity, sleep, and heart health. Employ apps to track your diet, stress levels, and sleep quality. For more in-depth insights, consider gadgets like body composition scales or HRV monitors.

Regularly review the data these tools provide. Look for patterns that might indicate inflammation, such as poor sleep, increased heart rate, or sudden changes in body composition. Share this information with your healthcare provider to tailor a personalised plan for managing inflammation.

7.4.Community and Support: Finding Your Tribe

When you decide to follow an anti-inflammatory diet, you might be taking a significant step towards better health. This diet focuses on foods that reduce inflammation in your body, which can help with conditions like arthritis, heart disease, and even some cancers. However, making such a change isn't always easy. This is where finding a community of like-minded individuals, or your "tribe," can make a big difference.

Foods to Include:

Fruits and Vegetables: Rich in antioxidants, these foods help reduce inflammation. Think berries, leafy greens, and colourful vegetables like bell peppers.

Whole Grains: These provide fibre and nutrients that can help lower inflammation. Examples include brown rice, oats, and quinoa.

Healthy Fats: Omega-3 fatty acids found in fish, nuts, and seeds are known for their anti-inflammatory properties. Olive oil is another excellent choice.

Lean Proteins: Fish, chicken, and plant-based proteins like beans and lentils are great for maintaining a healthy diet.

Spices and Herbs: Turmeric, ginger, and garlic have anti-inflammatory benefits and add flavour to your meals.

Foods to Avoid:

Processed Foods: These often contain unhealthy fats and sugars that can increase inflammation.

Refined Carbohydrates: White bread, pastries, and sugary drinks should be limited.

Red and Processed Meats: These can contribute to inflammation and should be eaten sparingly.

Trans Fats: Found in many fried and packaged foods, these fats are harmful and should be avoided.

The Role of Community in Dietary Changes

Making dietary changes can feel overwhelming, especially if you are doing it alone. This is where finding your tribe becomes crucial. A community can provide support, encouragement, and shared experiences that make the transition smoother and more enjoyable.

Emotional Support

Changing your diet can bring about a range of emotions. You might feel excited about the potential health benefits, but also frustrated by the limitations and challenges. Having a group of people who understand what you're going through can be incredibly comforting. They can share their stories, offer tips, and help you stay motivated when you're feeling down.

Practical Advice

A community of individuals following an anti-inflammatory diet can be a treasure trove of practical advice. From sharing recipes to suggesting substitutes for your favourite inflammatory foods, these members can help you navigate the everyday challenges of this lifestyle. For instance, they might have tips on how to make a delicious meal with anti-inflammatory ingredients or where to find the best deals on healthy groceries.

Accountability

When you're part of a community, you are more likely to stay committed to your goals. Knowing that others are watching your progress and that you are part of a supportive group can encourage you to stick with your diet, even when it's tough. Whether it's through a social media group, a local support group, or friends and family, having people to answer to can boost your perseverance.

Shared Learning

Nutrition science is always evolving. Being part of a community means you have access to the latest research and can learn from the experiences of others. Someone in your group might have discovered a new anti-inflammatory food or a cooking technique that could benefit you. Sharing knowledge helps everyone grow and maintain a healthy lifestyle.

How to Find Your Tribe

Finding a community that shares your dietary goals doesn't have to be difficult.

Here are some ways to connect with others:

1.Online Forums and Social Media Groups:

Platforms like Facebook, Reddit, and Instagram have numerous groups dedicated to healthy eating and specific diets. Joining these can connect you with a vast network of people worldwide.

2.Local Support Groups:

Many cities have health-focused meetups or groups that gather to discuss diet and wellness. Check local listings or community centres for options near you.

3.Workshops and Cooking Classes: These can be

a great way to learn more about the anti-inflammatory diet while meeting people with similar interests.

4.Friends and Family:

Sometimes, the best support comes from those closest to you. Share your goals with friends and family and see if anyone is interested in joining you on your dietary change.

BONUS

<u>*30-Day Meal Plan*</u>

<u>Week 1</u>

<u>Day 1</u>

Breakfast: Greek yoghurt with berries and a sprinkle of chia seeds.

Lunch: Quinoa salad with mixed greens, cherry tomatoes, avocado, and a lemon-tahini dressing.

Snack: Sliced apple with almond butter.

Dinner: Grilled salmon with steamed broccoli and sweet potato.

<u>Day 2</u>

Breakfast: Smoothie with spinach, banana, blueberries, and almond milk.

Lunch: Lentil soup with a side of mixed green salad.

Snack: Carrot sticks with hummus.

Dinner: Chicken stir-fry with bell peppers, broccoli, and brown rice.

Day 3

Breakfast: Oatmeal topped with walnuts, flaxseeds, and a drizzle of honey.

Lunch: Turkey and avocado wrap in a whole grain tortilla with a side of mixed fruit.

Snack: A handful of mixed nuts.

Dinner: Baked cod with quinoa and sautéed spinach.

Day 4

Breakfast: Whole grain toast with mashed avocado and a poached egg.

Lunch: Chickpea salad with cucumber, tomatoes, red onion, and a light vinaigrette.

Snack: Celery sticks with guacamole.

Dinner: Stuffed bell peppers with ground turkey, black beans, and brown rice.

Day 5

*Breakfast:*Smoothie bowl with mixed berries, granola, and a drizzle of almond butter.

Lunch: Spinach and mushroom quinoa bowl with a lemon-olive oil dressing.

Snack: Sliced bell peppers with tzatziki.

Dinner: Shrimp and vegetable stir-fry with a side of wild rice.

Day 6

Breakfast: Chia seed pudding with coconut milk and sliced mango.

Lunch: Grilled chicken salad with mixed greens, cherry tomatoes, cucumbers, and a balsamic dressing.

Snack: Fresh berries and a handful of walnuts.

Dinner: Roasted chicken with sweet potato wedges and green beans.

Day 7

Breakfast: Buckwheat pancakes topped with blueberries and a dollop of Greek yoghourt.

Lunch: Black bean and avocado salad with a lime dressing.

Snack: Cucumber slices with cottage cheese.

Dinner: Baked tilapia with quinoa and roasted asparagus.

Week 2

Day 8

Breakfast: Smoothie with kale, pineapple, and coconut water.

Lunch: Lentil and vegetable stew.

Snack: Sliced pear with a handful of almonds.

Dinner: Grilled tofu with sautéed bok choy and brown rice.

Day 9

Breakfast: Overnight oats with chia seeds, raspberries, and almond milk.

Lunch: Quinoa and black bean stuffed bell peppers.

Snack: Sliced tomatoes with basil and olive oil drizzle.

Dinner: Baked chicken thighs with roasted Brussels sprouts and wild rice.

Day 10

Breakfast: Greek yoghourt parfait with granola and mixed berries.

Lunch: Spinach and chickpea salad with a lemon-tahini dressing.

Snack: Apple slices with sunflower seed butter.

Dinner: Seared tuna with a side of roasted root vegetables.

Day 11

Breakfast: Smoothie bowl with spinach, banana, and flax seeds topped with granola.

Lunch: Turkey and avocado salad with a citrus dressing.

Snack: Baby carrots with hummus.

Dinner: Grilled shrimp with quinoa and roasted bell peppers.

Day 12

Breakfast: Oatmeal with sliced almonds, cinnamon, and a drizzle of maple syrup.

Lunch: Mediterranean chickpea and cucumber salad.

Snack: A handful of pistachios.

Dinner: Baked salmon with a side of steamed kale and sweet potato mash.

Day 13

Breakfast: Avocado toast on whole grain bread with a sprinkle of hemp seeds.

Lunch: Quinoa and roasted vegetable salad with a lemon-tahini dressing.

Snack: Sliced bell peppers with guacamole.

Dinner: Chicken stir-fry with snow peas and brown rice.

Day 14

Breakfast: Smoothie with spinach, apple, and ginger.

Lunch: Lentil soup with a side of mixed greens.

Snack: Fresh berries with a handful of walnuts.

Dinner: Grilled cod with a side of quinoa and roasted vegetables.

Week 3

Day 15

Breakfast: Chia seed pudding with almond milk and mixed berries.

Lunch: Quinoa salad with arugula, chickpeas, and a lemon dressing.

Snack: Sliced cucumber with tzatziki.

Dinner: Roasted chicken with butternut squash and green beans.

Day 16

Breakfast: Greek yoghourt with honey and sliced almonds.

Lunch: Spinach and turkey wrap in a whole grain tortilla.

Snack: Sliced apple with cashew butter.

Dinner: Grilled shrimp with brown rice and sautéed spinach.

Day 17

Breakfast: Smoothie bowl with blueberries, banana, and flax seeds topped with granola.

Lunch: Lentil and vegetable stew with a side of mixed greens.

Snack: Sliced pear with a handful of pistachios.

Dinner: Baked chicken breast with roasted Brussels sprouts and quinoa.

Day 18

Breakfast: Overnight oats with chia seeds, raspberries, and almond milk.

Lunch: Quinoa and black bean salad with avocado and a lime dressing.

Snack: Baby carrots with hummus.

Dinner: Grilled salmon with wild rice and roasted asparagus.

Day 19

Breakfast: Smoothie with kale, pineapple, and coconut water.

Lunch: Turkey and avocado salad with a citrus dressing.

Snack: Sliced tomatoes with basil and olive oil drizzle.

Dinner: Baked cod with quinoa and steamed broccoli.

Day 20

Breakfast: Oatmeal topped with walnuts, cinnamon, and a drizzle of maple syrup.

Lunch: Mediterranean chickpea salad with cucumber and tomatoes.

Snack:Fresh berries with a handful of almonds.

Dinner: Chicken stir-fry with bell peppers and brown rice.

Day 21

Breakfast: Buckwheat pancakes topped with blueberries and a dollop of Greek yoghourt.

Lunch: Black bean and avocado salad with a lime dressing.

Snack: Cucumber slices with cottage cheese.

Dinner: Seared tuna with a side of roasted root vegetables.

Week 4

Day 22

Breakfast: Smoothie with spinach, apple, and ginger.

Lunch: Quinoa and roasted vegetable salad with a lemon-tahini dressing.

Snack: Sliced bell peppers with guacamole.

Dinner: Grilled tofu with sautéed bok choy and brown rice.

Day 23

Breakfast: Chia seed pudding with coconut milk and sliced mango.

Lunch: Lentil soup with a side of mixed greens.

Snack: Sliced pear with a handful of walnuts.

Dinner: Baked chicken thighs with roasted Brussels sprouts and wild rice.

Day 24

Breakfast: Greek yoghourt parfait with granola and mixed berries.

Lunch: Spinach and chickpea salad with a lemon-tahini dressing.

Snack: Apple slices with sunflower seed butter.

Dinner: Baked salmon with a side of steamed kale and sweet potato mash.

Day 25

Breakfast: Smoothie bowl with spinach, banana, and flax seeds topped with granola.

Lunch: Turkey and avocado wrap in a whole grain tortilla.

Snack: Baby carrots with hummus.

Dinner: Grilled shrimp with quinoa and roasted bell peppers.

Day 26

Breakfast: Oatmeal with sliced almonds, cinnamon, and a drizzle of honey.

Lunch: Mediterranean chickpea and cucumber salad.

Snack: A handful of pistachios.

Dinner: Roasted chicken with sweet potato wedges and green beans.

Day 27

Breakfast: Whole grain toast with mashed avocado and a poached egg.

Lunch: Quinoa and black bean stuffed bell peppers.

Snack: Sliced apple with almond butter.

Dinner: Baked tilapia with quinoa and roasted vegetables.

Day 28

Breakfast: Smoothie with kale, pineapple, and coconut water.

Lunch: Spinach and mushroom quinoa bowl with a lemon-olive oil dressing.

Snack: Sliced tomatoes with basil and olive oil drizzle.

Dinner: Seared tuna with a side of roasted root vegetables.

Day 29

Breakfast: Greek yoghourt with berries and a sprinkle of chia seeds.

Lunch: Quinoa salad with mixed greens, cherry tomatoes, avocado, and a lemon-tahini dressing.

Snack: Fresh berries with a handful of walnuts.

Dinner: Grilled salmon with steamed broccoli and sweet potato.

Day 30

Breakfast: Overnight oats with chia seeds, raspberries, and almond milk.

Lunch: Lentil and vegetable stew with a side of mixed greens.

Snack: Sliced